YOU
CAN
THINK
YOURSELF
THIN

# YOU
# CAN
# THINK
# YOURSELF
# THIN

Transform Your Shape
with Hypnosis

*Ursula James*

JEREMY P. TARCHER/PENGUIN
a member of Penguin Group (USA) Inc.
New York

JEREMY P. TARCHER/PENGUIN
Published by the Penguin Group
Penguin Group (USA) Inc., 375 Hudson Street, New York, New York 10014, USA *
Penguin Group (Canada), 90 Eglinton Avenue East, Suite 700, Toronto, Ontario M4P 2Y3, Canada
(a division of Pearson Canada Inc.) * Penguin Books Ltd, 80 Strand, London WC2R ORL, England *
Penguin Ireland, 25 St Stephen's Green, Dublin 2, Ireland (a division of Penguin Books Ltd) *
Penguin Group (Australia), 250 Camberwell Road, Camberwell, Victoria 3124, Australia (a division
of Pearson Australia Group Pty Ltd) * Penguin Books India Pvt Ltd, 11 Community Centre,
Panchsheel Park, New Delhi–110 017, India * Penguin Group (NZ), 67 Apollo Drive, Rosedale,
North Shore 0632, New Zealand (a division of Pearson New Zealand Ltd) * Penguin Books (South
Africa) (Pty) Ltd, 24 Sturdee Avenue, Rosebank, Johannesburg 2196, South Africa

Penguin Books Ltd, Registered Offices: 80 Strand, London WC2R ORL, England

First published in 2008 by Random House UK
First American edition: Jeremy P. Tarcher/Penguin 2009
Copyright © 2008 by Ursula James

Most Tarcher/Penguin books are available at special quantity discounts for bulk purchase for sales
promotions, premiums, fund-raising, and educational needs. Special books or book excerpts also can be
created to fit specific needs. For details, write Penguin Group (USA) Inc. Special Markets, 375 Hudson
Street, New York, NY 10014.

Library of Congress Cataloging-in-Publication Data

James, Ursula.
You can think yourself thin / Ursula James—1st American ed.
p.      cm.
ISBN 978-1-58542-727-7
1. Autogenic training.   I. Title.
RC499.A8J36     2009                          2008054637
615.8'5122—dc22

Printed in the United States of America
1   3   5   7   9   10   8   6   4   2

BOOK DESIGN BY TANYA MAIBORODA

Neither the publisher nor the author is engaged in rendering professional advice or services to the
individual reader. The ideas, procedures, and suggestions contained in this book are not intended as a
substitute for consulting with your physician. All matters regarding your health require medical
supervision. Neither the author nor the publisher shall be liable or responsible for any loss or damage
allegedly arising from any information or suggestion in this book.

The recipes in this book are to be followed exactly as written. The publisher is not responsible for your
specific health or allergy needs that may require medical supervision. The publisher is not responsible
for any adverse reactions to the recipes contained in this book.

While the author has made every effort to provide accurate telephone numbers and Internet addresses
at the time of publication, neither the publisher nor the author assumes any responsibility for errors, or
for changes that occur after publication. Further, the publisher does not have any control over and does
not assume any responsibility for author or third-party websites or their content.

*To my wonderful husband, Phil, for always being there for me, and doing a great job of pretending to be sane. "Hey—I have had an idea . . ."*

# ACKNOWLEDGMENTS

My family (old and new) and friends for their love and for feeding me during this project.

Nicola Ibison at First Artist Management, Hannah Black at Random House, and the wonderful Lorraine Flaherty in Oz.

Thank you all for your support and help throughout this incredible year.

Also my thanks to Sarah at the Audio Workshop.

# CONTENTS

# LETTER FROM THE AUTHOR

READ THIS BOOK AND FOLLOW A SMALL PROPORTION OF the suggestions in it and you will definitely lose weight—without conscious thought or effort. In this book you will find a structured hypnosis program to guide you through effortlessly making long-term changes to your life. You will also find some of the latest research on *why* some people find it genuinely harder than others to maintain weight loss. I have also included easy-to-follow tips to keep you on track and motivated.

It is not just a poor diet and lack of exercise that make people fat. There are other factors too: lack of sleep, our environment, relationships with other people, and our personal history—to name a few. This book will help you understand the cause of your problem, and will give you the tool of hypnosis to help you help yourself—once and for all. This book is for you if you have ever *felt* fat—regardless of your weight. It is not just about weight control—but life control too. Obsessing about your body can damage your confidence and your relationships, and ultimately hold you back from the life you want. It is time to take back control.

By the end of this book, you will find a new, improved, fitter, healthier you, a person who feels in control of their life and who is strong and confident. You will also understand the real reasons behind your past weight issues, so you will be able to stop those things from affecting you.

It is time to stop hiding: time to have the life you want, the body you want, and the confidence that goes with them. Now all you have to do is read this book, follow the instructions, and listen to the self-hypnosis CD that goes with it.

Time to get excited . . .

*Regards, Ursula James*

# YOU
# CAN
# THINK
# YOURSELF
# THIN

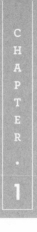

# PREPARING
# FOR CHANGE

## INTRODUCTION

Follow 20 percent of the suggestions in this program and you will lose weight and maintain that weight loss forever and without the struggle. This program prepares your mind-set, enabling you to carry out the changes that will make your weight loss permanent. It puts you back in control of your feelings and thoughts, so your weight-loss behavior will follow—automatically. Losing weight will become effortless, and when you reach your ideal weight you will be able to maintain it unconsciously.

The program in this book and in the accompanying CD uses a combination of coaching, self-hypnosis, and common sense. It also incorporates recent research that has radically changed our understanding about the problems of weight and obesity experienced in modern life.

It has an easy-to-follow structure in which you read, listen, and complete actions. The program is designed this way so that you will have access to the easiest way to learn the concepts and change your life. As I explained in my most recent book, *You Can Be Amazing*, each one of us has a primary (most easily accessible) way of learning new information. By including all the different elements in this program, you will be able to grasp the concepts easily, hear the lessons properly, and see what I mean when I describe how to make the changes in your life.

The nice part about learning in this way is that you do not need to think too hard about it. Learning should be easy, and it should be fun. When learning is at its most effective it is unconscious. By the end of this program you will have changed your attitude toward yourself, your weight, and your body image in a way that works best for you. It is not rocket science—but it *is* incredibly effective. The coaching suggestions in this book describe the Who, What, Where, and When of the problem, and the hypnosis in the CD provides the How—how to change your attitudes and to remain comfortable with your new ways of thinking, freeing yourself from past negative patterns.

## DEPRESSION

Anyone who has ever had to struggle with their weight has an idea of how miserable it can make you. These thoughts of dejection, of being "weighed down" by the feelings you have about yourself, can become almost impossible to describe. It is so easy for someone else to say "Cheer up!" when they do not understand how you really feel. We have a whole vocabulary that associates a state of mind with a physical sense of weight. We talk about *feeling low*, having *a load on our mind* or *a heavy heart*. The language of emotional weight is a comprehensive one. Feeling low psychologically and heavy physically are commonly connected. A major problem when dealing with weight control is being able to identify and tackle the psychological issues that caused the weight problem in the first place. Even though you feel better when you have lost weight, if you have not dealt with the underlying cause it will be a struggle to maintain your weight loss. Food will always be on your mind, and there will be a real and present danger of yo-yo dieting as soon as additional stress enters the equation.

This is why hypnosis is so significant in helping you to

change, by allowing you to deal with your history without consciously becoming aware of *why* you started the behavior. Hypnosis works by amplifying the natural ways in which we change and develop, thus making the changes accessible and long-lasting.

•     Certain foods can be very comforting. Stodgy food full of carbohydrates, which momentarily distracts you from your feelings, gives you a warm and cozy feeling inside that can often be confused with love. Once you have eaten too much of the food that comforts you, then the unhealthy cycle kicks in. You feel miserable, so you eat; then you feel guilty for eating, so you feel more miserable, and you eat more. All that stops here. In this program you first build up your confidence and feelings of self-worth, then go on to deal with the issues that got you into this mess in the first place (unconsciously if that is what you feel safest doing). The final act is to create a new future template for yourself that will be both flexible and have sufficient stamina to deal with whatever happens in the future. *It is time now to take control.*

Control is a fundamental issue around self-image and how we relate to food—control over what is going on in our lives. The less control we *perceive* we have, the more we reach for food as a way of controlling our internal environment. This habit developed over a lifetime of learning. The wonderful thing about the human mind, however, is that it only takes three weeks to completely eradicate habits and the associated mental connections that set those habits off. This will happen only when we recognize and accept, both on a conscious and an unconscious level, what we can and can't control in the world around us.

This acceptance of ourselves and our capabilities means also understanding what we cannot change. We cannot change someone else's feelings, for example. We cannot change the fact that we are getting older every day, or that we may have had some unpleasant experiences in our past. But once you have accepted these facts something fundamental does change within you. The stress associated with trying to change the world to exactly the way you want it will disappear. You will allow yourself to make mistakes and to accept that you can let other people help you. You can also accept that others will not always give you exactly what you want.

Being in control is also about being flexible and learning to accept that there will be times when things go wrong. How you deal with those times will give you the stamina to remain confident and on top of things. Being *truly* in control is about accepting that you are not always right and that you do not need to prove yourself in every area of your life. Control is about not only strength, but also flexibility and the ability to recognize that with this program *you can and will continue to change in a way that will work for you.*

Unlike many self-help books, this is tested theory. It is based partly on my own work with clients (mainly women) who came to see me with weight problems. I observed a number of common themes when women talked about *why* they felt they were overweight. I conducted further research and came across a review paper published in the *International Journal of Obesity* in 2007 that listed many of the reasons mentioned by my patients. I went on to discover that there is substantial research behind these "alternative" reasons for being overweight that my clients had talked about. Their reasons for having difficulties in getting control over their weight were valid ones—not excuses.

The reasons for weight problems listed in the review paper fell under ten headings:

- Sleep
- Body temperature
- Prenatal effects
- Fertility
- Age
- Drugs
- Pollution/chemicals
- Older mothers
- Your partner
- Smoking

I also found that there were other common factors identified by my clients:

- Stress
- Attitudes toward the self
- Attitudes toward food/eating
- Confidence
- Motivation
- Events in childhood

All of my clients had one thing in common: they felt as if they were not in control when it came to diet and exercise. They all *knew* that they should exercise more and eat less, and they had read numerous books about calories and fitness programs—but still they were somehow "unable" to do what they needed to do. So, before giving the usual suggestions for motivation for diet and exercise, I realized that these people needed to address their issues of control before working on anything else. This aspect of weight loss and healthy weight maintenance has been sadly overlooked in most diet and exercise programs. I discovered that the people I worked with had never been asked to look at their weight problems in these broader terms.

As you work your way through the program, you will learn how you relate to the world around you, recognizing what you can and cannot control. This will have a great impact on how you start to make the changes needed to *lose weight safely, effortlessly—and permanently.*

I have condensed my successful approach into this book and the hypnotherapeutic suggestions on the CD. The major difference between this program and others out there is that this is not primarily about diet or exercise. It is about recognizing and controlling the mental state that kicks in when we are told what to do and what not to do—and how it impacts on the way we treat ourselves.

By the time you have finished reading this book and working your way through the CD and the tasks, you will be a different person. The program will help you create a confident, healthy image that you will not only project to the outside world but that you will also *become.* However, before you get there, the hypnosis will allow you to understand what it was that got you where you are now so that you never slip back into old destructive patterns again.

When your unconscious reveals how you became the person you are, this will help you to visualize how your current moods and behavior will change, allowing you to picture clearly who you are going to become in the future. That future will see you free of your old destructive habits.

## WHAT IS HYPNOTHERAPY AND HOW WILL IT HELP ME?

There are three hypnosis tracks on the accompanying CD. Each one deals with a different time in your life. Track one concentrates on *the past* and how you became the person you are now. It helps you to recognize certain attitudes from the past that have had a negative influence on you and your relationship with your body. The second track focuses on *the present* and the ways in which you currently behave and feel. This will guide you through the practical, day-to-day steps you will make to change your negative patterns and create new, positive habits. The third and final track will help you to focus your mind on *the future* and what will be different in your life when you have made these changes. It will allow you to look forward to your new life in this future place. It is designed to motivate you, and to keep you on track with your newly created attitudes toward yourself, your success, and the world around you. The final track also has suggestions to help you deal better with stress so that *nothing and no one will ever be able to trick you back into the old patterns—no matter what!*

You may not be aware of it, but you have probably experienced hypnosis before. Hypnosis is most commonly recognized as a state of deep physical relaxation, with heightened mental focus. Whenever you get really involved in what you are doing, and it is something you enjoy, such as reading a book, watching a movie, or a physical activity like swimming, you will notice that you can become so absorbed in what you're doing that there seems to be no effort involved at all. This sensation can also occur when you are driving down a familiar route, and you make all the appropriate turnings *without any conscious effort on your part*. You are so absorbed in what you are doing that your awareness of distractions around you is reduced, and you concentrate completely on what you are doing, to the exclusion of anything else.

When you are in hypnosis, this is exactly what happens. Your body becomes so relaxed that you no longer pay any particular attention to it. Your mind becomes clear and can pay close attention to one thing at a time—and that is it. It is *not* a general anesthetic, and you *do* hear everything that is said to you. In fact, the state of being in hypnosis is very pleasant and relaxing. If you have ever meditated, or found your attention drifting while you had a massage, you will recognize this state. An interesting thing about this is that when you are *in this state you forget about food—in fact, you can forget about all the things that usually stress or bother you.*

*Hypnotherapy* is slightly different. It uses hypnosis to make previously agreed-on suggestions more acceptable and possible to the person in hypnosis. When someone goes for a one-on-one hypnotherapy session, it must first be decided what type and form of suggestions will be made in the hypnosis. If the hypnotherapist makes suggestions that were not previously agreed to, the person in hypnosis will immediately reject them—often waking themselves up in the process. This is why I have designed this program so that you will be prompted to do tasks that help *you* to create the suggestions. You will then feel safe and in control, and so get the full benefit of the CD tracks.

Some people are nervous about the idea of hypnosis because they think it is about letting someone else control and influence them. *No one* can make you do *anything* you do not want to do—ever. While listening to the CD you will be mentally focused and alert, and you will remember all of the suggestions that are relevant to you. In fact, you decide which of the suggestions are going to work best for you. There are three tracks on the CD, punctuated by a chime so you will not accidentally go from one to another. In this book you will be told when to listen to each track. You should allow around twenty minutes to listen to each track. Track one and two you listen to *only once*. Track three you listen to daily for twenty-one days, then afterward whenever you need extra support to keep you on track. I have designed this program to make it as close to a one-on-one treatment as possible. Suggestions are built in to the CD tracks to ensure that you will only take on board those that are safe, appropriate and relevant to you. So, when you come across suggestions that are not relevant to you, you will ignore them. In fact, you will only listen to and remember those that apply to you, and you will only register and respond to the suggestions that will help you to get what you want out of the program. This replicates a completely natural process that happens every day in our normal, waking lives. During an average day we are exposed to huge amounts of new information, but we connect only with information that will be useful to us and that is relevant to our lives. This brings me to one of the greatest ironies about this process: during hypnotherapy you will not be told anything that you don't already know.

When I talk about your conscious mind in this program, I am referring to the part of you that rationalizes and analyzes. Hypnosis works by getting your conscious and unconscious minds communicating effectively. It is well worth my reassuring you again at this point about the process. You will be in control while you are experiencing it—and the net result will be a positive one, because you are selecting suggestions from the book and the CD that will be the most useful and practical for you. You will discard all other suggestions, along with the previous version of you and its associated behaviors.

How, then, does this help you? Quite simply, there is a massive difference in the way you receive and accept information when you are hypnotized, and how you then go on to access and act on this information at a later date. When you are in a relaxed state, with nothing around to distract or disturb you as you listen to the suggestions, the information will be received and processed by the part of your brain that is involved in habitual and unconscious responses. That means that you will not need to think about changing your behavior—it will simply happen to you—naturally and effortlessly. When you are in hypnosis you are listening, and paying attention, only to the suggestions that make sense to you. You will reject any suggestions that are not helpful. This program is designed to take all the knowledge that you have about yourself and your relationship with food, and translate it into something that your brain can comprehend and start to unconsciously put into action. Using hypnotherapy this way works because you hardly notice that you are doing things differently at all—but you *will* notice the results.

## How the program works

As with *You Can Be Amazing*, this program is designed so that by reading through it, doing the exercises, and listening to the CD *you will unconsciously take on board suggestions in the most effective way for you*—with very little conscious or deliberate effort on your part. All you need to do to complete the program is to read through this book and, where prompted, either listen to a CD track or complete an action. The book will tell you how much time you need for each track or action, so you can plan more easily. The final track—*Future*—is designed so that you can listen to it whenever you feel that you need help to stay motivated.

Each person will read the book differently, will hear and interpret the suggestions differently, and will get different responses by doing the exercises. Each person's history and relationship with their body is unique, so each person's interaction with the information is different. You, too, will respond in a completely unique way to the program because you will be tailoring it to yourself and your lifestyle as you go through it. This is the main reason why this program is so successful. It becomes your own personal program, and the hypnosis ensures that the suggestions you are open to taking on board become well and truly fixed into your unconscious. When this happens, *nothing and no one can divert you from having the relationship with your body that you want.*

### How is this different from the other methods I have tried before?

The program's uniqueness lies in these three elements:

- It helps you recognize where your problems came from.
- It helps you create new, positive habits so you don't even notice that you are changing.

- It helps you create an image of yourself in the future that will become your "dream motivator."

*The book also has tips and hints throughout to guide you and keep you firmly on track.*

Finally, the main difference between this and any other program is the way it uses the state of hypnosis and, separately, hypnotherapy—the power of your own mind—to make positive suggestions that are safe, practical, and acceptable. It works because it works with you, in a way that will allow you to make the changes effortlessly. It is only when you look back on what you have achieved *three months after reading the book that you will really be aware of how much you have changed,* because in this time you will have built new habits into your life, and will see how much weight you have lost and how much better you feel about yourself generally.

Throughout the book you will find ACTIONS. Read the whole action through before doing anything. This way it will be much easier for you to carry it out and you will also know how long you need to complete it properly.

## How do I know this program will work for me?

There is a simple test you can do to see whether you fit into the profile of people who benefit most from this program. Take a piece of string and measure out a length you feel will be long enough to go around your waist exactly. Do this by eye only. When you have cut the length, see how accurate you were by wrapping it around your waist. I guarantee you will find that the string you cut is *much longer* than you thought it would be. When the problem of weight is a problem with your mind, rather than with your body, you will *feel* bigger than you are. This has a direct impact on how you carry yourself, how you dress, and how you behave. Also, if you are an emotional eater, feeling fat will cause you to eat more because you feel depressed. This will be dealt with later in the book, and with suggestions in the CD that will help you not only lose weight but also lose the attitude of failure. You will gain confidence *and* the body you have always wanted.

This program is designed to be simple. All the directions in the book are supplemented by hypnotherapy suggestions and motivation techniques designed to make carrying out the directions for change easy. You will not take all the suggestions on board—in fact you will be very selective and only take on board those that will work for you with the life that you have now. There are other suggestions in the CD tracks—ones that are not connected to specific directions in the book. These suggestions are designed to motivate you and focus your attention on what it is you want to get out of the program. Finally, there is another set of suggestions that run through the program designed to give you the confidence to make the changes you need—and, most significantly, to maintain them effortlessly.

## *The importance of feeling good about ourselves, and why it is sometimes hard to lose weight*

Having a weight problem is rarely simply a matter of eating too much and exercising insufficiently. This program is for people who have tried diets, exercise regimes, and classes, and are making themselves miserable by depriving their bodies of food. A weight *problem* needs more than a simplistic strategy—it needs the individual to change their mind about who they are and what they want out of life. This program is about discovering who you really are and taking control back of your life—not about restrictions and prohibitions. It is about the joy of food, and fitness and living life to the full.

Once you have completed the program, your thought processes will be altered in such a way that diets will become a thing of the past. By the end of the program you will have a level of control that will influence not only the way you think but also the way you feel and behave. Nothing will be able to trick or fool you into eating in response to false hunger *ever again*. Your relationship with your body and the world around you is key to this change, and taking on board positive suggestions about yourself on a deep, unconscious level will mean that the changes will be permanent and you will be sufficiently flexible to deal with your world and yourself as both change.

When I talk about alternative reasons for putting on weight, I am referring to all the factors other than diet and exercise that influence how we feel about ourselves and interact with the world around us. Our levels of interest in ourselves and how motivated we are to make these changes need to come from within, and until you create a healthy vision of your future self, change is not going to happen—and even if it does it is unlikely to give you everything that you want as part of that change, like becoming happier with yourself.

### How much of the program do I have to do for it to work?

Simply put, you do *not* have to follow every suggestion in the book, nor will you take on board anywhere near all of the suggestions from the CD. The best way to read the book is out of interest—rather than *trying* to consciously work at change or learn new habits. So *don't try;* instead let your unconscious mind do the work for you. If anything, *trying* makes it more difficult for you to make far-reaching changes because if we *try,* we are consciously aware of what we are doing, and the more we try, the easier it gets for us to start unraveling the changes. We start to talk ourselves out of the new and useful behaviors and back into the old, inappropriate ones. The fact is, we are wired to maintain the status quo; that is our *habit-ual* way of doing things, even if it is damaging.

For this reason, the hypnotherapeutic component of this program is instrumental in making the changes stick—permanently. Once your unconscious mind—the part of you in charge of habits—recognizes the new behaviors, thoughts, and feelings installed through the hypnosis, and you then *consciously* start to register the benefits of these new patterns, any effort on your part in making these changes happen will disappear. You will no longer have to think about what you are doing, because the newly installed patterns become second nature and *you will carry them out without any conscious thought or effort on your part. Easy.*

In some cases, you will not be registering new patterns of thought, feeling, or behavior, but reconnecting with ones that were natural and habitual to you *before* you learned the unhelpful ones. We can learn these behaviors in many ways, and I will talk more about this later in the book. For some of us, recognizing that we are not the only person in the world to feel this way or have this particular weight problem helps us to change ourselves. Having a weird relationship with your body is much more common than you might think—although women are often too scared to talk about it for fear of seeming self-obsessed or neurotic. That attitude stops right now—you are not alone—nor are you "mad, bad, or dangerous to know." By the end of the program you will have the control you want and need over your life and your body—and you will be able to recognize others who have also made this journey. These are strong, confident, sexy people. It is about time you became one of them. Something to aim for—don't you think?

So now we turn to the shape of this program. At varying stages in the book, you will be prompted to listen to the three CD tracks. You will listen to each track only once while working through the program. Remember, track three can be listened to more than once and will keep you on track after the program. There will also be actions to complete. You will be told how long to allocate to listen to the tracks or to do the actions. Sometimes you may leave the book for a few days before picking it up again. You will take this at your own pace. The first of the tracks is designed to look at anything from your past that is relevant to your relationship with your body, and nourishment, and to disconnect from the habitual patterns that have no place in the here and now. Additionally, it looks at giving you the confidence to deal with some of the elements of your personal history.

This book is not intended as a substitute for one-on-one therapy, and if you recognize through doing this program that there are some things from the past that you need to deal with in a more proactive manner, the program will give you the strength to go on and deal with them. You may notice that strong memories from your past keep coming up. These will be things that you unconsciously know that you need to deal with now. They will only come up as a result of the program if you are able to take action and deal with your past. I will describe the contents of the other two tracks when we get closer to them. You may feel you need more help than this program can give you. If this is the case I have supplied some web addresses (see p. 191) as a starting point.

# HOW DID YOU GET HERE?

IN THIS CHAPTER, I WILL TALK ABOUT THE DIFFERENT versions of you that exist and how they came about. To explain this, consider this question: Have you ever experienced that feeling you have when you've done something and you feel you weren't yourself? For instance, "I don't know what came over me—I didn't intend to eat the whole package of cookies."

There is irony here, because in order to feel in control and "remove" the unhelpful versions of ourselves that are responsible for overeating, we need to make our conscious and unconscious communicate in a way in which they ordinarily do not. When I talk about unconscious I am really describing the part of you capable of going on autopilot—the part of you that controls waking, sleeping, digestion, and so on.

First and foremost for some people, your overeating habit protects you from an emotion that you couldn't deal with at a point in your life.

One example of how this can happen is the teenager who becomes very stressed at the thought of upcoming exams, and as a way of coping with the stress starts eating lots of toast. As she starts to get bigger, she begins to buy clothes to "hide" in and develops a habit of wearing big, baggy sweaters. After a while she starts to associate the clothing with relief from stress, and begins to put a baggy sweater on *automatically* whenever stressed.

The important thing to note here is that the overeating and the baggy sweater disguise go hand in hand. She needs to throw out that baggy sweater as much as she needs to stop overeating. This program will unconsciously help you to give up these old and harmful habits.

However, if you don't deal with the original trigger, i.e., in this example, stress, the "self" starts to send out messages to get you to take notice—and these messages take the form of symptoms. For many women these symptoms are expressed as feeling out of control in relation to food. Until you deal with the emotion stored by the protecting "self," you cannot process your history, and the symptoms remain live. In the second hypnosis track you will be able to safely communicate with this self and the emotion held by it, in such a way that it will directly disconnect you from whatever triggered the symptoms. You will then be back in control of your behavior and will be able to create new, healthy ways of relating to food and your body. It takes three weeks before the new responses filter through fully and become your new habits. A wonderful part about using the hypnotherapy in this way is that you remain completely in control throughout. You are aware of what is happening—and by the end of the process, you have gained control over the areas of your life where you had little or none before.

The teenager described above ate when she was stressed. Think about your overeating. When do you overeat?

When you are emotionally healthy and stable and no longer eat in response to "false hunger" (more on this later), you will literally be at one with yourself and you will then be in control of your eating habits. You will eat healthily when you need to and not in response to emotional triggers.

The many eating responses you have developed during your lifetime are, in essence, "emotional snapshots." Just as a photograph of you is an image frozen in time, and the image in the photo remains the same as you grow and develop, so the overeating person is a captured emotion that stays as it was when it was created, even though *you* may develop emotionally over time.

Here are some examples: the tired mom with small children who absentmindedly finishes off her children's food even though she is not hungry; the office worker who has a long commute and without thinking treats herself to a pastry on her way home; the working mother who habitually orders calorific takeout on Fridays. Long after their life has changed, some people continue the damaging behavior *automatically.* This program is designed to make you aware of any of your behaviors that have gone on autopilot—the behaviors that—if you described—you'd talk about them as if *someone else has taken over. Once you have recognized the selves or the mood that takes over, and dealt with their triggers, you will never feel out of control of your eating habits again.*

As you work your way through the program, these unhelpful "selves who take over" will fade and disappear, making room for one clearly defined, emotionally stable, and healthy self. By dealing with your negative moods and emotions and finding that one confident and emotionally healthy self by the end of the program, you will succeed in losing weight. You will also have your moods and habits under control so that there is no longer the temptation to sabotage all your good work, because the real *you will be in control from now on.*

When I have worked one-on-one with clients—and I am talking more about women here (although this applies increasingly to men)—I have identified that the selves get created in response to strong emotions and get refined in response to specific moods. By identifying when and how these selves came into existence, and recognizing the moods that triggered them, you can identify which components are useful, and which need to be discarded.

This process occurs in CD track 1—*Past*. It will take you along an emotional "time line." This in turn will allow you to go into your past safely while remaining completely in control of your experience. You will only go back to the times that are relevant to helping you create your new self. You will find what works for you and discard what doesn't. The best part is that you do not need to be consciously aware of how these changes are happening. You will, however, notice that you start to feel less stressed and emotional and more positive about situations in the here and now.

## TRUSTING YOUR UNCONSCIOUS MIND

Thinking about different versions of yourself might seem a little schizophrenic, but in actual fact, all of these characters were created in response to specific situations experienced by you, and all have behaviors that are designed to protect you.

It may not seem as if they are working in your best interests sometimes, especially if they are damaging in some way— bulimia or binge eating or drinking, for example. However, it is worth realizing at this point that any quick way in which your unconscious mind can move you away from an emotional state that you cannot deal with, can, with repetition, go on to register as valid. Even if the behavior causes harm in some other way, if it takes you away from feeling the *immediate* upsetting emotion, then this new, potentially harmful behavior can register as useful. If repeated over a period of three weeks, the new behavior will become habit and you will find that you have a different problem from the one you started with. The original reason for needing to shift your emotion has been masked, while the new behavior settles in for the long haul and creates a space for itself in your habits. This leaves you busy dealing with your inappropriate strategy and at the same time unable to deal with the reasons behind it.

Please note—this program is designed to help you move forward. It does so by allowing your unconscious to make the mental connections that will help you to recognize that you can take control in the here and now, and ultimately, that is all that matters. You cannot change your history, but you can change your relationship with your past. This program will help you to let go of the damaging effects of your history so you can move on in an emotionally healthy way

## CASE | HISTORY

**HARMFUL HABITS**

Christina was a student at a university. She was doing well but became really stressed when it came to her exams. Every day she would walk by a bakery on her way to lectures, and every day she found herself saying: "I am not going to have a doughnut. I am being good." Then the exams got closer, and she became more and more stressed. The bakery suddenly became irresistible, and she found that when she had eaten the doughnut she momentarily felt better—less stressed. Every day from then on, she would have a doughnut on the way to school. In the end she didn't even think about it; it became automatic. Even after the exams she was still doing it. It had become a habit. "I didn't even enjoy it in the end," she observed.

Christina came to see me when she was in her final year, and she was so obsessed about her weight that she couldn't concentrate on studying. I noticed that she always wore the same clothes, black and baggy. She described her clothes as her "fat clothes—something to hide in." I worked with Christina and helped her recognize the connection between stress and food, then taught her some relaxation techniques and worked on breaking the bakery habit. This involved simply taking a different route to lectures for three weeks—enough time to break the habit. Once this had happened, I encouraged her out of her "fat clothes" and into something more colorful and flattering to her shape. Immediately she looked slimmer, and her confidence soared. She quickly started to lose weight.

Once Christina was able to identify the connections between her trigger mood—stress—and the habit that had developed around it, she soon took control. The clothes she wore when being the stressed/fat person went in the bin—never to be replaced. She passed her exams and has never fallen into the stress/eat cycle again because she has control over her moods and deals with stress before it affects her.

and succeed in getting to your healthy target weight once and for all.

The hypnotherapeutic process in this program is very effective in helping you take control of your relationship with your body. The process effectively retraces your neurological steps, without the emotional associations, allowing you to find the most effective ways of changing. In the same way as your behavior seems to happen without you thinking, so the hypnotherapeutic process develops without conscious thought. All you have to do is to retrace your steps, and this can be done while relaxing in hypnosis.

The hypnotherapy will do the work for you as soon as you start to *trust this part of your mind to do its job properly.*

## What can cause these destructive moods to emerge?

The medical definition of trauma is *"any injury, whether physically or emotionally inflicted."* Most people, especially if they have experienced traumatic life events, become afraid to look back into the past to identify the root of their problem behavior. This is often out of a fear that they will be made to relive the disturbing events in their past or, even worse, to discover something that they did not already know about. It is important for you to understand the ways in which the brain registers information. Memories only become damaging when the effects of those memories have not been fully processed. We have all had things happen to us in the past that we'd rather not relive. With this process you will *not* relive them. You will only revisit the *emotions* associated with your memories as a way of helping you to move forward— and you will only do this if *you have not already processed these emotions.* So you may feel an emotion during the hypnosis, but you will probably not remember the event it relates to.

What is traumatic to a child may not be traumatic to an adult—so the event you have been so afraid of looking at will seem very different when you view it with adult eyes. Also, when you stop thinking about something that happened, the memory of it will fade naturally. As the memory fades, any emotion that is part of that memory fades too. This is a natural process. An example of this is hearing a particular song that reminds you of an ex-boyfriend. When you first heard that song after splitting up, you would get upset. Then, as time went by, the sadness connected to the song faded—so in the end you could listen to the song without it upsetting you or reminding you of past events.

With this program you can look back on events in your past as part of this process and know that you will only access a memory if it is significant in helping you change and get better, and as and when you do, you will be safe and in control. Memories cannot harm you—only the way in which you react to them can. This program is designed to help you to safely access just the active parts of memories that will help you to move forward—and only in a way in which you can deal with them.

Whether or not you buy into the idea that there is a separate part of your thought processes that operates without your conscious awareness—the unconscious—you cannot deny that there are many physical functions and behaviors that you do without thinking. Breathing, your heart beating, even learned skills such as the ability to drive a car: all of these functions and processes operate without your conscious thought. It therefore follows that there is a part of our mind that controls all of these things—and can operate without conscious involvement—even in our sleep. This is the part of the mind that is actively engaged in this process, and we call it the unconscious mind.

As I've said, out of all the suggestions in this book and within the CD, you will recognize that only *some* of them will apply to you. Those that do apply to you, you will take on board and act upon. This works in a similar way to the 80/20 rule, known as Pareto's principle. To paraphrase this rule, 20 percent of what we do is vital, and 80 percent trivial. The only problem with this is recognizing which of the changes you are making are vital to making your new behavior long lasting and which of them are trivial. During the three weeks after completing the program you will find that only some of the new behaviors remain with you. These are the ones that you will have reinforced in your sleep—and therefore made your own. So there is actually no need to *think* about what you want to take on board, or what you *think* will work for you— your unconscious mind will make that decision and *act only upon the suggestions that feel right for you.*

As a result, by the end of the program you will notice that real changes have occurred, but if you try to analyze what you are doing differently, you will feel as if you are only doing a small proportion of the program. You may also notice that *you are feeling much better generally, better about yourself and the world around you, and more able to let go of the things that used to bother you.* This is how it should be. There are two facts that you might find interesting at this point: one is that the suggestions in the hypnosis will encourage you to pay attention to what is working for you, and to disregard what will not realistically fit into your life, and second, you will have taken on board many of the suggestions for inner change—i.e., a change in attitudes, without ever being aware that this has taken place.

## Why did these moods stay around?

These strong moods that stick with you are part of your stuck past. When stressed or traumatized by events and unable to deal with them at the time (perhaps because we are too young or the event is too upsetting), our unconscious mind copes by creating a "mood" in which we feel we are someone else, whose function it is to deal with specific memories so we can get on with life.

What you are experiencing is different and unhelpful moods. Before you can get rid of them once and for all, I will explain how they arose in the first place by telling you a little about the psychological theory of dissociation. Dissociation is a "splitting off" of a part of "self" in response to a trauma. This part is then identified by certain characteristics or behaviors and is triggered in specific situations. Recent literature classifies dissociation as a defense mechanism occurring in response to situations where the individual has no immediate control. This could be triggered by a combination of factors, like being tired, run-down, and stressed, and then having something significant happen—not necessarily unpleasant in itself—such as moving or having a baby. The person may then be left with the feeling that they cannot cope with what is going on in life. Then it is as if a part of you separates off to deal with the event. It takes between three weeks and three months of disturbance for the "part" of you to be created that will respond to the trigger situation. The newly created "part" will then take over and act out a behavior, such as bingeing on food, that serves the purpose of turning those feelings of helplessness into other types of feelings. The behaviors are like signals from the split-off part of you that is trying to cope with events, forcing you to pay attention.

To understand *why* this happens, it is important to understand the nature of pain as experienced by the brain. Bear with me on this; there is a point to this digression.

If you are experiencing intense physical pain, the stress and irritation of work will no longer register in your brain at

## CASE | HISTORY

### UNDER PRESSURE

Gillian was a journalist and new mother. She really enjoyed her work and was very happy being a mom. There were times when she felt she wasn't a good enough mother or progressing fast enough in her journalism career, but she recognized these feelings as normal. When her baby was eighteen months old, Gillian was offered the role of subeditor with a prestigious magazine. She took the job, and rapidly noticed that the pressure of work was amplifying her feelings of inadequacy both as a mom and in her professional role. Added to this, her daughter became ill, and the manageable pressure she had felt before now became overwhelming.

Gillian started to binge on rich, "treat foods," something she had started doing when she was studying for her exams at school. Her feelings of inadequacy subsided, taken over by an immediate feeling of being too full. She started to make herself sick, and then she felt guilty and revolted by herself. She described the event of bingeing and purging in this way: "I couldn't stop myself—once I started to think about it, I became obsessed, and could do nothing else until I had satisfied this need—it was as if someone else had taken over."

that moment. Seems obvious, doesn't it? It is the same mechanism that kicks in for people who self-harm. Your brain can only experience and process one type of event at a time, and it will choose the most intense and immediate event to pay attention to. This is why, when you binge, you cannot *feel* the emotions that triggered that behavior in the first place, and because this part of you is carrying out the behavior on an unconscious level, you feel out of control—as if you cannot stop yourself from doing it. The binge only stops when you have forced the brain into paying attention to a different, more immediate sensation—that of being completely stuffed full of food. The brain then moves its attention to dealing with this immediate problem, and the mood that triggered the binge is forgotten. The dissociated self then hands control back over to you, and you then are left to deal with the aftermath—as well as new negative feelings of disgust and nausea.

The most important point to recognize here is that each one of these moods were "made" and evolved over a period of time until they took up a space in your life. Each mood, effectively, has its own personal history, its own reason for being— and it is only by understanding its stories and recognizing the purpose it was created to fulfill that you can give it (and yourself) permission and assurance to change. This is where the hypnosis part of this program really comes into its own.

You will, like most people reading this book, have tried to

analyze and understand your behavior and your relationship with food. You may even have a good idea of how these moods came into existence and the purpose each one fulfills in your life. However, when you listen to the first CD track, you will get to meet these moods on an *emotional* level. You will meet them in your unconscious mind, the part of your mind where they have control, and your mind will be able to work with them so they can hand control back to you.

How it works is that each mood triggers a behavior. When you go into that mood, you "act out" specific thought processes and behaviors. It is at this point that you feel out of control and a binge can occur. The binge stops only when the mood has been turned into something else, often disgust, guilt, or exhaustion. Following the hypnosis, you will be able to identify and then control the moods that created the behaviors. All you really need to know at this stage is that your behaviors are created in response to a trigger, which has its own needs—needs that, up until now, you have indulged or avoided with food.

When you tried in the past to change your eating and exercise habits, you will have noticed that you found yourself thinking about food even more than before. Your inner voice was giving you reasons *not* to exercise, *"It's too cold today," "I can't find my swimsuit," "I really ought to telephone X"*—until you found you had talked yourself out of exercise. Now you have all the time in the world to think about the food you were trying so hard *not* to think about. "I may as well put the kettle on, then," your inner voice says, innocently, knowing full well that when you do that you will also have a cookie or make a sandwich to go with it. Once in this pattern, the regime of diet and exercise is broken, and we begin to feel bad about ourselves, which then can trigger another bout of eating and more negative self-talk—all reinforcing the old, inappropriate habit.

When you experience the first CD track and its hypnotherapeutic suggestions, you will meet your other selves on their own territory, your unconscious mind, and you will communicate with them with the purpose of having them hand control of these habits and behaviors back to you—the conscious and aware you. As I have already mentioned, it will take about three weeks before you are fully in control of these behaviors, but you will *notice the differences in your behavior immediately.* As the weeks go by, the new habits you want to install will take over as replacements. Also, because these new behaviors are much more healthy and appropriate for you, they will be stronger than the old, negative habits, and, *from this point in time, no matter what mood you are in, you will be in control of your eating habits.*

## SLEEP

I include sleep here because it can be both a reason for putting on weight and a reason we might find it difficult to lose weight. You need to have good sleeping patterns for the program to work properly. Also, if you had had good sleep in the first place, you would have naturally processed any problems, avoided the mood that triggered the "not you" behavior, and been able to move on.

Poor sleep can dramatically affect our eating patterns and behaviors. There have been a number of studies linking body mass index (BMI) to hours of sleep. These studies show that people who sleep less than seven hours a night are likely to have a higher BMI than those who sleep more. In fact, for those who sleep less than six hours it is higher still, and for those who sleep less than five, even higher. We all know that some people seem to need more sleep than others, but there are also other relevant factors that affect sleep patterns. For example, when people are very overweight, their sleep can be disturbed by snoring or discomfort as a direct result of the weight. Disturbed sleep also upsets the metabolism, obvious to anyone who has worked shifts or does a lot of long-haul traveling, or new mothers who have to get up throughout the night to feed a young baby.

Poor-quality sleep also affects our eating habits and cravings, as the sensations of sleep deprivation can be misinterpreted as hunger. These include feelings such as dizziness, light-headedness, or a vague emptiness.

The solution to this lies in regulating your sleep patterns to help maintain healthy leptin levels and allow your metabolism to return to a healthy and appropriate tempo. If you are currently in a situation where work or home life is forcing you into unusual sleep patterns, then you will absorb the suggestions in the first hypnosis track that are designed to help you gain as much benefit from sleep as you can until you are able to regulate your patterns.

One thing I would like you to consider is that if your unusual sleep patterns are due to anything other than a new baby, the longer you go without sleep, the more strain you will suffer. We can all cope with unusual or disturbed sleep for short periods of time, but when it is long-term it can be quite damaging to your health. Your ability to concentrate will be reduced, so accidents will happen more often. You will feel more out of control, and your moods can become volatile, so your relationships with people around you will be affected, as will your ability to make decisions. If you are in this situation, consider changing jobs or lifestyle. Many people lose weight *without any apparent effort* when they leave a job, a relationship, or an environment where they were not happy. If you find that impossible to contemplate, remember what I have just said about lack of sleep affecting your ability to make decisions.

My final point here about sleep is to reiterate that sleep is essential for this program to work effectively. When we sleep, we move through different phases, most of which are rest phases. There is one specific phase of sleep, however, that has a more significant function. That is REM (rapid eye movement) sleep. We go through a REM cycle approximately every forty-five minutes during sleep.

Studies of brain activity during this phase of sleep show that we appear to be actively processing information, and using both imagination and memory. When we are starved of this type of sleep we become forgetful and irritable. This program utilizes your REM phase to transfer what you learn from reading this book, doing the actions, and listening to the CD into the unconscious part of your mind, where you can start to act on it as a new sequence of behaviors. The wonderful part about doing it this way is that your REM sleep acts as a form of mental rehearsal, so that when you are awake and you go into the trigger situations you will feel as if your new behavior is the most natural thing in the world. After twenty-one nights of sleep, when the program is completed, you will have allowed your REM phase to process everything you need for long-term change. Don't worry—I have put lots of suggestions into the hypnosis tracks, and you will always be aware of which suggestions you are choosing to take on board. You will, perhaps, be surprised at how *you find yourself responding to situations around food and your self-image in a different and much more comfortable way.*

## DAY-TO-DAY STRESS

I have devoted a whole section in this chapter to stress because how we deal with it dictates whether we ultimately succeed in losing weight and maintaining weight loss. And it is often because we are not able to deal with the stress of events appropriately that our unhelpful moods were created.

Stress results in fat retention, bloating as a result of water retention, bulking up through tensing of muscles, *and* giving you an appetite for sugar. Am I painting a clear enough picture for you here? Stress not only causes you to feel fat, but to be fat and become fatter as you eat in response to it. To break this stress/eat cycle you first need to recognize that it is happening.

Your patterns are unique to you. You may be a midafternoon snacker or someone who reaches for a glass of wine in the early evening as soon as you have put the children to bed. Whatever your patterns, I have created a series of suggestions in track two of the CD. These suggestions are designed to act as a pattern breaker. You will become highly aware of your negative food/stress behaviors, and as the next three weeks go by, you will become more and more aware that you are thinking before responding, then responding differently.

It is important to ensure that you do not fall back into old, negative patterns of behavior. When you get stressed, it is almost as if the brain switches to a default setting for behaviors and thoughts, and the result is that you can very soon find yourself yo-yoing in terms of both your weight and your feelings about yourself.

As you know, sleep patterns will affect your stress levels, so in track two I will make some direct suggestions to help you sleep better, and wake feeling refreshed, relaxed, and ready to approach the day.

I keep a notepad on my bedside table, which I use to write down things I need to do the next day. By doing this you may find that you sleep better, as you no longer have those things on your mind. There is nothing worse than trying to go to sleep while thinking "I must not forget . . ." You can guarantee that it will disturb you. And a funny thing about your memory is that it tends not to register negatives, so it will hear "I must . . . forget," wiping out the "not" in the process. Giving yourself the suggestion to *remember* rather than *not for-*

*get* is a useful aid at any time of day when you want to re-member something. Tell yourself "I will remember," and take out the "must" as well. You will find that your ability to recall improves when you remind yourself with positive language and without the pressure of the word "must."

# PAST TIMES AND HOW
# THEY STILL AFFECT YOU

IN THIS CHAPTER I WILL FURTHER EXPLAIN HOW YOUR behaviors are responses to emotions from your past that you were unable to deal with at the time. You will also understand your habits and behaviors in relation to food and eating, and discover how they belong to your other self that we spoke of in Chapter 2. By understanding and getting that self back under conscious control you will have control over your eating habits forever.

In this chapter you will be prompted to listen to the first of the hypnosis tracks, called *Past*. You will listen to it only once, and you will be able to hear and remember everything that is being said to you while you are in hypnosis. There may be times when your attention wanders, and that will be fine. The most important thing for you to know is that you will be in control throughout. Once you have listened to the *Past* track, you will have made the unconscious connections with your history that will help you get back in control. *This will be strengthened in your REM sleep over the next three weeks, so you will notice the changes more and more over that period of time.*

This chapter is all about clearing the way for change by looking into your personal history and reviewing the times and places when your moods were created. I must emphasize again that this program is not designed as a substitute for therapy if you have serious issues that affect you on a day-to-day basis. This program *is* designed to give you enough confidence and self-awareness to reduce or remove the *effects* of your past in a way that will specifically help you to cope better in the present and create a more healthy and positive future. By working through the program you will not be going on a comprehensive tour of your personal and emotional history—but you *will* become secure enough to access any emotions that have become triggers for current inappropriate behaviors, such as comfort eating or binge-purge patterns. It is like turning around in a nightmare to see the monster that is chasing you. It is never as bad as you feared—and once you *have* looked, you have control.

When you go back in time through memories and associated feelings to identify what, if anything, is relevant to the way you feel today, it is essential to remember two important points about memory. These apply not only when you use hypnosis for recall, but also when you sift your memory for information regardless of the method that you use.

First and foremost is that your memory is not an accurate representation of events that happened to you. It is very selective. Second, it will present the events through the filter of your conscious awareness. In other words, your recall of events will be changed by the knowledge that you have about yourself today. We make mistakes. We fill in the gaps about what we do not remember fully. It is not that we are *lying*. It is just that we are attempting to make sense of our past in the safest way for us. This sometimes means that simply by trying to recall an event, we forget our role in the event, or something that will completely alter our understanding of the event. This is why going into your past to find the *solution* to your problem can sometimes be a pointless exercise and, in some instances, positively damaging. Accessing memories to understand yourself better and to recognize what factors from your past have made you into the person you are today can be a very helpful part of self-healing. Analyzing the events and trying to make sense of something that may have been completely *senseless*, however, can result in you fixating on the past instead of moving on in a healthy way. By experiencing the suggestions in the *Past* hypnosis track on the CD, your unconscious will begin working on the events from the past and putting them into their proper place in your memory. This means you will no longer be bothered by your history in the same way, your emotional response to that history will fade, and you will take back control of your eating habits—forever.

This program is structured in a very specific way to ensure that you will always feel (and be) safe to make this journey into your past. No suggestions are made to "lead" you to specific times and places in your memory, so there is no danger of acquiring a "false memory" by using the program. I spend time in the next CD track—*Present*—building up your emotional and psychological stamina so that you will be ready, open, and prepared to deal with the associated emotions that may come to the surface as part of the process.

Your memory will only give you access to information that it feels you can deal with *at this time* and, most important of all, it will only give you access to information about yourself that will be *relevant* to helping you change your current feelings and behaviors in a positive way. I have no doubt that at some time in the past you will have reviewed your history, either by talking with family members or friends, or even through therapy. You may have even done this alone. Which-ever method you have tried, most of you will have, at some point, looked back as a way of understanding how you devel-oped certain responses and behaviors. The frustration arises when you think you have a very good idea of where things originated but *still* cannot change how you think and feel in the here and now.

So, whether you have reviewed your history already, or are afraid to go there, this first CD track will ensure that you feel safe with what you can learn there about yourself. If you do not feel that your past has any relevance to your present, be-cause you either have dealt with it or feel that you have no need to deal with it, the program covers this too. You are com-pletely in control in the hypnosis, and you will access only emotions and knowledge that will help you to make the changes that you want.

When anyone looks into their past for a therapeutic pur-pose, it should be for one reason, and that is to gain insight to help them to move forward. The first hypnotherapy track will help you look into your history to make sure that there is nothing holding you back. It is designed to help you to change your relationship with your history, so that from this point in time you will start fully living in the present and begin to get a clear image of where you are going in your future. You can-not change the past; no one can. You can, however, change your *relationship* with the past in such a way that it will no longer hold you back. Changing in this way will also help you to move forward in an emotionally balanced way.

## CHILDHOOD TRAUMA AND STRESS

Over the years there have been countless studies on childhood trauma and its impact in adulthood. Only recently has a direct link been established between physical or sexual abuse at a young age and heightened levels of C-reactive protein in the blood. The significance is huge. C-reactive protein is linked to, among other things, heart disease.

Stress at an early age changes the body's biochemistry to such a degree that as an adult the individual's system will react to events in ways different from the system of someone who was *not* traumatized. It is no longer a matter of linking childhood trauma with adult maladaptive behavior. Now science has established a direct link between childhood events and adult biochemical reactions. For anyone who has yo-yo dieted as an adult this link may help you understand why you changed your *behavior*—but you did not change the way you *feel* about yourself, and as a result you responded in a child-like way because this is all that the "self" knew. It is as if you grew up, but the part of you with the problem did not—it remained a child. So when you got stressed, you responded by eating, just as the child used to.

## Why does overeating help someone who was traumatized in childhood?

Simply put, overeating overloads the brain to such an extent that it momentarily pushes all other memories out of your mind. Your system can cope with only a limited number of events at any one time, and there is a hierarchy of needs. Again, I will use pain as the example.

First, pain is processed in the same brain region, regardless of whether that pain is physical or psychological. Second, our brain needs to decide what to deal with first. The brain categorizes the pain into types, according to whether it is high grade or low grade. You cannot react to two different events at any one moment in time—for example, if someone makes you laugh when you are having an argument, you cannot stay angry. The result of the brain's need to pay attention to one type of pain at a time means that it will pick the acute physically *consuming* pain before anything else, as it recognizes that this is the most important and the one to deal with first. So, if you break your leg all other types of pain that you *would* have been experiencing at that moment (such as feelings of stress) are pushed out of the brain to make way for dealing with the urgent physical pain situation. There is a direct parallel here with overeating when pained by personal stress. People can overeat until it *physically hurts*. When this happens, they can no longer process (or even register) the much lower-grade stress/pain that triggered the overeating in the first place.

To recap, people who have a predisposition to a poor stress response because of the events of their childhood will be excessively affected by stress in their adulthood. If food was used as a means of comfort for that individual as a child, then food will be used in the same way in adulthood. The problem comes when the adult system fails to respond to the food in the same way, and so the individual keeps eating and eating until the discomfort and pain of being really full block out the capacity to *feel* the emotional pain that triggered the bout of comfort eating in the first place. This then becomes a habit because it has a payoff, and the behavior then becomes unconscious and increasingly difficult to control.

When you overeat you overload the system with work— kicking off biochemical processes to deal with the overload and as a result pushing the emotional pain from your immediate awareness. You are too involved with dealing with the effects of the food to register the emotional pain.

## CASE | HISTORY

**AFRAID TO EAT**

Ella experienced some very traumatic events in her childhood. As an adult, she developed some curious behaviors—one of which was that she had become obsessive about the types and quantities of food that she ate. She only ate by the clock—and became very distressed if she could not eat her food at the appointed time. She was well below average body weight for her height, and her periods had stopped as a result. Ella had psychiatric and psychotherapeutic treatments that helped her to understand where her problems came from, but this didn't help her to take control of them. This added to the stress she was already feeling.

While I was working with Ella, she told me that one of the most traumatic incidents she remembered from childhood centered around a Sunday lunch, where she was pulled away from the table for doing something wrong (she never did know what) and beaten so badly that she had to be taken to the hospital. Thereafter, Ella associated food directly with pain and with being out of control of events.

When Ella had to deal with food, she felt compelled to control as much as she could, so that "the event from her childhood would never happen again." Logically and consciously she knew that it wouldn't—but when it came to food she felt as if "someone else was taking over, and she couldn't stop herself from obsessing." I taught Ella how to hypnotize herself and negotiate with the "self" who took over at mealtimes. After a while, Ella gradually started to—in her own words—"come back to the table—to attend meals"—something that, until this point, had terrified her.

## What is false hunger?

False hunger is the name given to the "butterfly" feeling you get in your stomach when you get upset and then eat in response to it. This can be made worse if you are really stressed and as a result become light-headed and dry mouthed, all part of the stress response but easily confused with the effects of hunger.

How does this confusion come about? Well, when we are young, we are absorbing huge amounts of information from the world around us, and it is not always easy to recognize which of our learning is going to be useful to us and which is potentially harmful. If we are well balanced and have enough reference points around us that enable us to distinguish good learning from bad (parents, friends, siblings, etc.), then we naturally identify what lessons will be useful to us, and we reinforce this ability as we grow up. These techniques then become habitual, and we can forget about them as our unconscious mind takes charge. An example would be learning how to behave near the edge of a cliff, or what to do when we learn how to ride a bike. Once an action has become unconscious it gets keyed in to a part of our mind where it will be stored until needed. We learn much more quickly if there is some stress caused by the potential danger of getting it wrong. Therefore, a little stress can help us "fix" a memory securely into the unconscious part of our mind. Imagine, for example, that as a child you are in a situation that scares you and you have all of the stress responses described above (dry mouth, butterflies in your stomach, etc.), then someone gives you something to eat to calm you down. If this happens often this can become a learned response. So, among all your useful learned responses, you will have one that associates food with relief from negative feelings—in other words, false hunger. By the end of this book you will have learned to deal with stress appropriately and will also have connected properly with the part of your mind that allows you to register real hunger. You will have broken the connection between emotion and food once and for all.

## YOUR BODY IS NOT THE ENEMY

How often have you heard someone say, *"I hate my body"*? If that someone is you, then this section of the book is going to be crucial in helping you to change your relationship with your body.

First, let's look at some of the reasons *why* you might have this attitude, and see how the hypnosis is going to help you to change those negative feelings. It is vital for me to stress at this point that by using this program to move forward and change your feelings about your body, you do not need to understand where these feelings about yourself came from, nor will you have to think consciously about your history.

For the most part, people who have body issues are fairly self-aware about the origins of those issues, in the same way that most individuals who have ever dieted are experts on calories and the different types of diets available. What I am getting at here is the fact that it is not enough to know where your problem originated (or suspect that you know—more about that later). Nor is it enough to have all the facts on *how* to change your diet and lifestyle. Fundamental to long-term change in attitude about your body is the reduction (and ultimately the removal) of the negative emotional connections with certain aspects of your history, and the creation of new, positive connections with your present and your future. You have to like yourself and your body enough to make that change happen, and to turn those lifestyle choices into a permanent feature of your life.

## How is this going to happen?

In the first CD track you will find suggestions about your past, and, more significant, your relationship with your history. Without being aware of it, each one of us develops habits around the way we think, feel, and act. For the most part we do not register that these are just habits. It then becomes easier to believe that these thoughts, feelings, and behaviors are what we *are*, not what we *do*.

The hypnotherapeutic suggestions in CD track one will help you to separate out your unhelpful habits from those that will be useful for you as you change. They will also make it much easier for you to recognize when you are doing things purely for the sake of it. The suggestions are designed to register as soon as you hear them; then over the next three weeks—twenty-one nights of sleep—your unconscious mind will continue to work on the suggestions. By the end of the three weeks, you will have completely taken on board only the ones that will work *for you*. (Remember, tracks one and two you listen to only once, track three, every day for twenty-one days and thereafter whenever you need a top-up.)

Before we can set about getting rid of your destructive moods/emotions, you will have to work with them. First, your unconscious needs to recognize why these moods and emotions originally came about, and to deal with this if you have not already done so. Second, you need to negotiate with them—because these feelings need to be acknowledged and given space within you. Then you will have to recognize that these are all aspects of *you* and have served a purpose—that of protecting you when, perhaps, you were not able to protect yourself in any other way. *All of this communication described above will be unconscious.* At no point will you become aware of this process, as it will happen during the hypnosis and at night when you enter the REM state, when your unconscious mind works on the events of your life and helps you to understand them in a way that will be useful and healthy for you. Sometimes, this means helping you to forget what happened. Some people experience events in their lives that are so awful, there will never be a way of making sense of them. For some people the only way to survive and move forward is to forget what happened. Amnesia of traumatic events is not uncommon, and it is there as a protective mechanism. I want to reassure you of this: if you have had things happen to you in your life that fall into this category, *you are not going to awaken memories as part of this process.* This process concentrates on the here and now, and will only access memories that are

## Hypnosis | SESSION 1

**THE PAST**

Now we come to the first of the three CD tracks; it should be listened to only once. This first track will work with you on your relationship with the past. All of the suggestions in this track are designed to help you let go of inappropriate thoughts, feelings, and behaviors, any of which could have held you in the trap of yo-yo dieting. Not all of the suggestions will be directly relevant to you, and such is the wonderful power of the unconscious mind that you will ignore any of the suggestions made that are not relevant to you. This will leave your thoughts clear to take on board only the suggestions that work for you.

In this track you will hear a suggestion to go into your past, to a time and a place that is relevant to your relationship with food. The important thing to stress here is that you may not consciously remember what that event is—and it is not important for you to do so. The purpose of suggesting that you do go to this time and place is to recall the neurological connections that were in place moments before. How does this work? Well, if you think about it, before you had a problem, you had a perfectly normal and healthy response to food—even if you do not consciously remember one. So, the objective is not to get at a memory—but to make a connection, the healthy connection. The hypnosis is then used to make that connection "live" and reintegrate it into the present.

Rest assured: You are not going to remember an event—but you may remember an emotion. If you do, you will allow yourself to experience this feeling—safely and for the last time. You will feel better as a result. One of the most wonderful things about hypnosis is that it allows us to become aware of the connections in our mind that already exist, and reconnect the healthy, appropriate, and normal responses that we need to move toward our goals.

| Time Needed to Complete Action |  | 20 minutes |
| --- | --- | --- |

**ACTION**

Track one: *Past*

Go to the toilet if you need to.

Turn off your phone.

Choose a time and find a place where you can be undisturbed. You can sit down or lie down, as long as you are comfortable. Do not cross your arms or legs; allow them to relax.

If you wear glasses, take them off.

Close your eyes.

Now listen to the first track on the CD, called *Past*.

When the track is over, sit or lie still for a few moments to make sure you are fully reoriented.

Remember: if anything happens that needs your
attention while you are listening to the CD, you will
become fully alert and able to respond.

If you want to write down anything that you thought of
or felt as part of listening to the hypnosis track, do so
now. You can review it again tomorrow before
continuing with the program.

I suggest that once you have listened to the hypnosis
track, you give the program a rest for today. You can
pick it up again tomorrow.

associated with events from your past if you have not dealt
with them in a way that will help you to move forward. More
important, it will only access them if they are relevant to moving you forward, and if your mind feels safe and comfortable
enough to deal with the repercussions of change. Helping
you feel in control of your life is a big part of this program. You
will, of course, be safe and in control throughout this process,
and in the hypnosis especially. You are driving it—and you will
keep yourself completely safe throughout.

You have now completed the first section of the program.
You have become aware of things from the past that have had
an impact on your weight. Now, by listening to the first CD
track—*Past*—your unconscious mind can work on putting
your past to bed, properly. Any feelings or behaviors around

food stemming from the past that are inappropriate in the present will now be processed. At night, when you dream, your unconscious mind will sift through everything you have learned and start to mentally file away anything that is no longer useful for you.

# BECOME AWARE
# OF THE PRESENT

WE NOW MOVE ON TO THE *PRESENT* SECTION OF THE program. This is covered in the next three chapters. It ends (like the last section) by listening to a CD track to put all this knowledge to work—unconsciously. In this chapter, I will help you become aware of things in your present that have an impact on managing your weight.

The first section of the program was the hardest part of all—it gets much easier from here on. After completing the first section, some people prefer to take a break for a week or so before continuing with the book. The choice is entirely yours. If you are feeling quite emotional as a result of what you have allowed yourself to access during section one, then I recommend that you do take a break before reading the next chapters of the book. We nearly always underestimate the time it can take to let new learning sink in properly, and feel compelled to rush on to the next task. This is counterproductive. You need to take time to let change filter through to your unconscious mind, where it can be fully taken on board. This allows any changes to be permanent. Also, it will allow you to be flexible enough to accommodate any stress resulting from the unexpected effects of change. Always allow yourself to work through the program at the pace that suits you best. Remember that in your sleep and, particularly in the dream phase of your sleep, you are continuing to process information anyway. *As you have made new connections with your past—connections that will now allow you to move to a more positive phase of life—you need to start noticing the changes as they happen. Focus your attention on what is different* in your life now and give yourself time to let it sink in before moving through the next section of the program. If it is too soon, put the book down and come back to it when you feel ready to continue.

Over the next three weeks the full effects of connecting with your history in a more healthy and normal way will take effect. Remember that when you were listening to the last CD track you were allowing yourself to clear out negative connections with your history, and to create new and positive ones to strengthen you. At no point were you changing the past—but you were changing the ways in which you relate to it. It is important to recognize that although you are a product of your history you can, by changing the way in which you react to your past, move forward in a healthy and more normal way. At no point did you need to consciously recall events from your past—the hypnotherapy in the first track allowed you to access only the emotional bridges with your history that used to carry you over into old, negative patterns of thought and behavior.

You are now at a point in the program where you are strong enough and ready to move on. Before you do, however, you need to ensure that at no point in the future will you trick yourself into reverting to any of these old patterns. While doing the program, your mind will identify the form that some of these patterns take, so you can register them both consciously and unconsciously as a way of making sure that you are in control from now on.

## MEMORIES OF FOOD

For everything that happens to us, a stronger memory will form if there is emotion associated with it—good or bad. That is why it is easier to remember what you were doing on your birthday or Christmas than to recall what you ate for lunch four days ago. Our emotions produce distinct biochemical changes in the brain that allow us to "fix" such an event more deeply than others. This is a very primitive function that is designed to help us remember people, places, and events significant to us so that we *know* how to respond and do not have to waste time relearning the response time and again. Therefore, we learn much more quickly if there is emotion involved in any event. This is, for the most part, useful to us. However, when that emotion triggers a pattern of behavior that is unhelpful—such as overeating to comfort ourself—this becomes a problem. Because this response is unconscious, the easiest way to change it is through hypnosis. The hypnosis helps you get through to the part of you that can make the change happen—and because it is unconscious, we do not need to *do* anything to make it happen. At no point in the program will you need to *work* on the changes. The hypnosis tracks will make sure that you take on board *only* what will work for you to lose weight, and you will notice as the days go by that you are thinking more positively and getting on with the things that you already know will help you to lose the weight forever.

When you are listening to the hypnosis tracks, the first set of suggestions is designed to help you relax. Relaxation is a state in itself, with associated emotions that have nothing to do with your relationship with food. So, as you listen to the CD tracks you start to become more relaxed. The suggestions are then made so that you can experience future times of celebration or sadness *without* the conditioned response of overeating—in other words, you will become more relaxed about food and about yourself. In fact, on an unconscious level you already know this. The suggestions on the CD will make the connections you need to be able to act on this knowledge, safely and unconsciously, by transforming this connection with food and emotion into one that works more constructively for you.

So, how can our memories affect our eating habits? Well, quite simply, when we go into an emotional state, either negative or positive, we trigger the behavior associated with it, and if that behavior involves overeating, then that is what we do *without thinking about it*. If you take a step back and look at it, the eating is not the problem—the problem is the emotional state from our past, and overeating occurs because of the fact that your *response* is an unconscious one. Hypnotherapy will work in two separate ways to help you deal with this, and I will cover both in track three of the CD. For now, all I would like to do is explain how these emotional triggers can affect you, so that *you can start to become much*

## CASE | HISTORY

**HAPPY TIMES**

Donna went out drinking with her friends on her eighteenth birthday. She drank large amounts and when she got home, she made herself some Stilton on toast—something she would never ordinarily eat. After that, a good night out wasn't a good night to her unless she finished it off with her treat food.

In this example, Donna had formed a connection between celebrating and Stilton on toast. If she had been sick as a result of eating it instead, she would not have formed the connection. In trying to recapture the happy feelings from her birthday party, she was using the Stilton as a physical reminder. She did this for twenty-two years without even being aware that that is what she was doing. She cut out the Stilton on toast and lost seven pounds in three months—without making any other changes to her lifestyle.

*more aware of them and be able to take direct, conscious control* before the negative eating pattern takes hold.

The key is breaking the link between an emotional state and an unconscious behavior, whether that emotional state is a good one or a bad one.

## POINTLESS EXERCISE

If you are a gym bunny, and love your time on the treadmill, do not bother reading this section. If, on the other hand, you are a bit of a gymphobic, read on. I do not like exercise. I never have. I also know that I am not alone in this. I associate the word *fitness* with sweaty gyms and women with scary sinews, swigging huge amounts of water out of enormous bottles. I associate the word with discomfort and effort—two things I want to avoid at all costs. Unless I am doing something constructive or learning something new, I find that I get bored very quickly. From asking my clients similar questions, I found that this was a familiar problem. The key is first, find an activity that you actually enjoy; and second, incorporate other activities into your day that count as exercise.

Have you ever looked at the muscles on a housecleaner (a good one, I mean)? Mine had the muscle tone of an Olympic athlete, and, allowing for good genes, she put it down to the fact that she was cleaning houses four days a week. Ironically, I feel I have worked very hard to afford a cleaner, but when my cleaner left, I took over her job. Oh, boy, did it make a difference. Apart from the enormous feelings of satisfaction that it gave me, I quickly noticed my body toning up. I genuinely enjoyed cleaning the house and, because there was an end product, I didn't mind doing it. Even ironing burns calories, and as for gardening, it is great exercise.

The other activity I rediscovered was walking. Not only is it wonderful exercise for the body, it also allows your brain to take a break and, while you are doing it, you find all kinds of ideas start to flow. You can let your mind wander, and it is a brilliant way of getting rid of the irritations and stresses of the day. I incorporate a twenty-minute walk into my day wherever I am (except when on holiday, where a walk from the pool to the deck chair is sufficient). If I am really irritated by something, or want a more involved workout, I go for a walk along Oxford Street. If you want an exercise that will tax both your brain and your body, try getting through the shopping crowds on a Saturday. All that ducking and weaving will ensure that you are quite exhausted by the time you get home. You will find your own way of incorporating activity into your daily life. Go and play in the park with your kids, or walk the dog—borrow one if you have to. Laughter burns up between 2 and 31 calories per minute—and you should be doing this at least once a day.

When I work one-on-one with people who are depressed about their weight, one of the first things I do is prescribe a fast—and a tonic. Yes, I know I said that I didn't recommend fasts—but this is a news fast. No newspapers, no TV news, and no online news. No news at all. When you are feeling down, seeing death and destruction only makes you feel worse. The sky is *not* going to fall if you do not know exactly what is going on in the world—and if something is really important, let someone else tell you about it. Avoiding the news stops additional unnecessary pressure from coming in. I never read the newspapers when on holiday. That's when you really start to relax. Fast from news, and start taking the tonic. The tonic I prescribe is comedy. Laughter is wonderful stuff. The medical profession is now catching on to its benefits—not only in reducing the effects of stress but also in increasing our immunity and all sorts of other potential benefits. Stop taking life so seriously—you will live longer and enjoy it more.

So, in conclusion, my tip is you don't have to exercise to get fit. Exercise for that purpose alone can be boring. Instead, have fun in a way that leaves you breathing heavily and pleasantly tired and you will keep it up when you see the benefits. Use your imagination to find ways of going out there and getting moving. I have made some suggestions in track three of the CD to help you to do just this.

## TEMPERATURE

The good news is, there is a way of burning calories with no effort at all. You will even be environmentally friendly at the same time. Thanks to the wonderful innovations of air-conditioning and central heating, our bodies no longer have to work as hard to stay cool or warm. Mildly interesting, you might think, but what has this got to do with weight control? When you are in a room around 81°F, your body is considered to be "thermoneutral"—in other words, it is burning zero calories maintaining temperature.

Think about it logically: by making your body work harder to maintain a comfortable temperature you will burn calories. Studies on women have shown that by turning the heating down by 9°F (from 81°F to 72°F), their bodies consumed 239 calories *more* per day. That is the equivalent of .05 pounds of fat. All this benefit comes from simply turning the heating down. This is just one example of what I mean when I talk about the small but significant changes you can make. If you turn down the temperature in your home (do it gradually, so that no one else in the household even notices), you are making a change that will in turn make your body work harder. If you find yourself shivering occasionally, great—it means your body is being made to work. When your system has to work harder, you not only start to burn more calories but also are forcing a metabolic change—a small change that, when added to all the other tiny changes you will make, will give you the healthier, fitter metabolism that you have always wanted. Not only that but you will also save money on your fuel bills and help the ecosystem. Go on. It takes a few moments to do—so do it as soon as you can!

A cooler brain works more efficiently too. By turning down the temperature at home it will help you to get rid of that fuzzy-headed morning feeling. That is not to say you have to be cold—but the average temperature in homes in the UK has increased by 9°F in the last thirty years—so turn down that heat and make your body work that little bit harder.

## NEVER GO HUNGRY

A common mistake to make when trying to lose weight is to associate weight loss with having an empty, grumbling stomach. In fact, if you take a straw poll among women who have had weight problems, you will find the consensus belief is that they are only going to be able to lose weight when they start to get this feeling. This is *completely* wrong. The moment your stomach starts growling—and you become consciously aware that you are in need of food—it has already sent out unconscious signals to set your body into *famine alert* mode. Never, ever allow yourself to get empty. When your system gets into this mode, it is acting as if there is no food available, and therefore it will take steps to hang on to the fat in your body. Your metabolism will slow down, and that's when losing weight becomes really difficult.

The practical key here is to eat little and often; have healthy, low-calorie snacks on hand; and drink *lots and lots* of water. With this program, the suggestions made in the second CD track will create a new habit, so that you will be able to do this in the future without even thinking about it—instead of allowing yourself to get hungry. This way you will never feel as if you are on a diet or depriving yourself. *You will feel completely healthy and normal.*

## FAILURE IN THE PAST

When we decide to make a change of any kind to our lives, the first thing that happens is we unconsciously start to sift through our memory to help us imagine what it will be like when we do. This works well when we have been successful in making that change before—but works against us when we have not. In this case, if you have tried to lose weight before and *failed*, then this is the memory that you will base your future on. If the memories you find yourself focusing on are ones of failure, then you are creating an image of yourself failing in the future as well. We begin the creation of our futures using our memories of the past. This is why people yo-yo diet. They slip into the patterns from the past *unconsciously*—without even thinking about it. The hypnotherapeutic suggestions that you experienced when you listened to the first track on the CD worked on breaking this pattern, and changing your attachment to your past memories to help you create new images for the future.

With the hypnosis I will help you look forward to new ways of responding, instead of always looking back to how you have responded in the past. This will allow you to imagine a new self instead of recalling an old self. I will go into more depth about this later, but for the moment it is worth pointing out that imagining and remembering use the same area of the brain—so by keeping this area occupied with a positive future you are less likely to fall into the negative patterns of the past.

## NEGATIVE IMAGES

This brings me neatly on to the subject of images, and how we use our imagination and memory to create them—often going about it in a negative way. When most people diet, they think about what it is they *don't* want to do or to be. "I don't want to be fat," "I don't want to eat as much food anymore." These are the self-suggestions that bind. The problem with them is that when we suggest what we do *not* want, the brain has to create an image of the unwanted thing first, and then try to wipe it out. This is counterproductive.

Let me give you an example. You decide that you are not going to have the slice of cheesecake that you have just put into the fridge; instead, you are going to save it for later.

When you tell yourself this, your brain creates an image of the cheesecake and even which shelf it is sitting on to be sure it recognizes what you are referring to. Now you are thinking about the cake—and once this happens, your body starts to respond to the cake based on your memories (I like cheesecake), and you start to salivate. The battle is now lost, and the image of the cheesecake will not leave until you satisfy the physical process that you started by *not* trying to think about it.

So, to make suggestions that work, you have to deliver them in a positive way. In all of the hypnosis tracks I describe positive images (for example, an image of yourself looking fit and healthy) and I use positive language throughout (suggesting what you do want, not what you do *not* want). This way you will always be clear on what is being suggested to you.

Using positive language will become part and parcel of the suggestions that you are going to give yourself each day. Being positive about what you want requires a shift in your mind-set, but it is one that you are more than capable of making. As usual in this program, there is no need to think too much about this. The hypnosis suggestions throughout all three tracks will help you get into the positive self-talk. Also, as you start to notice the positive changes happening, your confidence will increase, and positive self-talk will become a fixed habit—one that you no longer notice.

# MOODS

# AND HABITS

THIS CHAPTER IS ABOUT FEELINGS, AND HOW THEY AFFECT you and what and how you eat. The purpose of this chapter is *not* to analyze your current patterns, but to help each person recognize that childhood patterns brought into adulthood can be transformed into ones that will be more useful in achieving and maintaining a healthy weight for life.

We see here how normal and healthy mood changes (like feeling angry or stressed out) can become exaggerated and potentially undermine your control over your weight and body image.

I am referring here to what can best be described as mood swings—dramatic changes in mood that can seem like an over-reaction to events you are trying to deal with at that moment. When it happens, you may feel as if you have little or no control, and that then takes you over. When it *is* over, you feel drained and often bad about yourself. You recognize that this behavior is out of character—but feel at a loss to control it.

Destructive mood swings occur for a number of reasons, and it is worthwhile looking into them now so you can better understand what can kick off a binge. Being able to take a step back and take control of your moods and the events that could potentially trigger the binge, long before a habit gets a chance to form, is really important. Habits that have already formed will be worked on in the CD.

This is the point in the program at which you are going to start moving from a focus on your past, and how it influences your behavior, to the present, and how it relates to your problem. By learning to *take control of mood swings now,* you will prevent old destructive patterns of thought and behavior from pushing you backward. Do not underestimate how strong habits can be. Even when you have taken control of the trigger for a mood swing (for example, when you work through unresolved feelings about a past situation, and understand *why* you are doing something in a particular way), you are still left with the associated habits and patterns in the here and

---

## CASE | HISTORY

**MOOD SWINGS**

Aisha was manager of a small company. She got little support from her immediate boss, and there was no one on her level to discuss work with. She felt lonely and isolated. On a particularly stressful day at work she had to deal with three separate unpleasant incidents. On her way home, she "treated" herself to a burger at the station—even though she knew that she was going to eat later anyway. Once home, and after eating her usual evening meal as well, her partner made one small comment that ordinarily she would have found harmless. This time she exploded in a temper. Without thinking, she ran upstairs and made herself sick—hoping to purge herself of the feelings of giving in to the burger. She then felt physically ill, as well as guilty for overreacting to her partner's comment.

This developed into a habit—and the relationship became very rocky as a result.

After two intensive sessions, Aisha decided to manage the life events that stressed her out in a more appropriate way, and separately worked on breaking the habit of binge/purge. Three years later, she is still in control.

---

now. In the next section of the program, which comprises the following three chapters, you will learn how to take control of the mood swings and the associated habits. Don't worry too much about applying this information to yourself. It is enough for you to read about it. The hypnotherapy suggestions in the CD will allow you to process and personalize it, so that only the parts of the program that are relevant will be accepted, and acted upon, by you. I will prompt you when it's time to listen to the next CD track.

Now I want to talk about something that you have started to address in section one of the program: the connections between your current moods and responses to situations from the past. I refer to these as emotional bridges, which allow you to effectively make connections that would not otherwise be made. The result of the emotional bridge effect is that you start to respond to the normal day-to-day events in an exaggerated manner. You are overreacting to what is in front of you, but without the capacity to take a step back and understand how you got so emotional. The feelings of being out of control become a problem on their own, and you start to dread the situations that seem to set you off. The simplest events can then become a problem—creating their own stress as you start to dread losing control.

## STRESS

Earlier I mentioned a research paper that linked childhood events with physical problems experienced in adulthood. The research shows how constant stress at an early age induces abnormal levels of inflammation in the gut. This becomes interesting when you consider why the body creates swelling. It is a response to pain, or the anticipation of pain. So now you have a model—a possible explanation—of why some adults are prone to bloating. Simply put, if they experience physical or psychological pain, their body will respond by swelling. As with the bloating caused by exposure or intolerance to certain types of food, it is an unpleasant and uncomfortable feeling. A feeling that, if we are already body-obsessed, will cause us to *feel* fat. Bloating and swelling can come and go, but once we have associated them with the tightness in our clothes that results from this problem, we may feel much heavier than we actually are. There are a number of gut-related conditions, IBS and Crohn's disease among them, that have been identified as becoming much worse when the individual is suffering from stress. Our stomach reacts when stressed, and for people who have conditioned themselves to eat as a way of changing feelings, this stress will increase the desire to eat.

So, rather than trying to control what and how you eat, as you have in the past, this program is designed to help you react to stress, whether past, present, or future, in a much more positive and healthy way. Once you have control over *how* you react to stress, your gut will get a chance to learn a natural and healthy response. In the future you will be able to deal better with any situation and without reacting by overeating, allowing you to eat better and digest properly. All of this you knew, if not consciously, at least on an unconscious level. The problem was that you only really registered it when it was already a problem, i.e., when you were already in the stressful situation and reacting to it with your old habits.

You can use the suggestions given in the hypnosis to help relax you and to reconnect with your body's natural and healthy responses to stressful situations. Using something like self-hypnosis, which will help you to take control of your response to stress, will help you to react better to stress generally. Even more important, you will be able to predict which situations in the past would have bothered you, and therefore to take control *before* you react.

If you do suffer from stress, using the *please yourself time* (explained fully later in the book) will become significant for you in taking control of how potentially stressful situations affect you. Taking time out to care for yourself will allow the effects of the stress to be diminished and so enable you to deal with stress much more effectively. The result is less bloating and inflammation and fewer times of *feeling* fat. Dealing with your stress and taking time for yourself will have a much greater impact on how your body reacts to food than you might initially realize. Taking time for yourself will also send out messages to your unconscious that it is okay to put yourself first—a really important message in making the changes you want a permanent feature in your life. Do this properly and these new habits will stay with you regardless of what is happening in your life.

## Stress treats

Have you ever said to yourself, *"I have been so good today—I deserve a piece of cake/glass of wine"* (insert your favorite mood-altering food here)? Do you recognize this? I bet most of you are familiar with this phrase even if you have never actually said it out loud. It can happen when the children are in bed, and it has been a long day—or when you have had a particularly unpleasant encounter with someone at work—and this little voice pipes up, *"Go on—you've been good—you deserve it,"* and a battle of wills commences. The battle of short-term gain (having your treat) versus long-term benefit (not overdoing it) begins with the other voice reminding you, "A moment on the lips—a lifetime on the hips." Oh, boy, do I hate these pat phrases. The more stressed you are, the more loudly and clearly the voice tells you, *"Just have what you want!"*

You can equate these two voices to those of a child (who has no idea of consequences and just wants instant gratification) and an adult (who can see the results of their actions). When your strong self emerges as a result of this program, your need to reach for the cookie jar (because that is what it is, really) will diminish. Two things will help you with this. First, the hypnosis itself is designed to relax you, in all three tracks. When you are more relaxed, you respond to stressful situations better and more appropriately, so breaking the habitual connections between feeling stress and eating. Second, when you have yourself back under conscious control, you are responding as an adult in the here and now and no longer with the childlike response that came from your history.

The connection between eating food as a response to stress and the negative feelings that follow becomes a vicious circle for some. But by taking your feelings back under control, *you will eat only in response to true hunger.*


## BINGE AND PURGE

If you have ever eaten to the degree that you have made yourself deliberately sick or taken laxatives to get rid of the food, your relationship with food has moved into a different zone.

If you eat to the point of disgust, and don't particularly care what it is that you eat, only that you must get something into your mouth, then you are responding to a very different need than hunger. If none of this relates to you, then skip this section. If it does, please pay attention now, because this part of the program will be key to your long-lasting change. Binge-purge cycles can be symptomatic of much deeper psychological problems, but they can also remain as habits long after you have resolved the issue that kicked them off.

If you have ever been in this binge-purge cycle, you will recognize that there comes a point when you literally cannot stop yourself. It feels almost as if you are on autopilot and someone else has taken control. In effect, someone has: an unhappy and stressed version of you. This other version of you or "self" only knows one way of dealing with stress, and that is to block it out with food. If you do have this pattern, and it is purely a habit now, you will respond very well to the suggestions in the second CD track, on which you will hear suggestions to take back control of the part of you that binges. This is a part of you not from the past, but one that exists in the present. These suggestions are all about taking back control in your life—the purging is only a symptom of your feelings of being out of control. Again, if this does not apply to you, you will blank out the CD suggestions that relate to it.

As I have said before, this program is not a substitute for therapy. If you have not dealt with the reasons behind your binge-purge behavior, you will need more help than this program can give you to eliminate your problem for good. You will be able to identify this clearly in the three months after completing this book. If you are still reacting to the old triggers, seek therapeutic help. I have put some phone numbers and addresses at the back of this book to give you a place to start. Regardless, you will have much more control by completing the program—and you *will* feel better. For some people, this program may be a means to an end and not the end itself. But even if it does not complete the job for you, it will help move you forward and give you the confidence to resolve your problem once and for all.

## Sexy shoes

A good friend of mine (who just happens to own a shoe shop) told me that "English women dress for their dogs, Italian women dress for their men." I am not saying that this is true, but it does strike a chord with me when it comes to footwear. Comfort over style is fine, but nothing ruins a good outfit more than a dodgy pair of shoes—or worse still, sneakers. I am of the belief that sneakers belong in a gym—and you won't see me in either! When I am out and about and I see (or hear) a pair of high-heeled shoes, and I look up to see the wearer I will usually see a confident person. Remember the *Sex and the City* phenomenon, when Jimmy Choos and Manolo Blahniks were talked about as if they were characters in their own right. High heels are sexy. They elongate your body—and raise your bum. They also make you much more aware of how you stand and walk. This is not to say that you have to wear them all the time (although I do know some women who do, and are perfectly comfortable in them as a result), but wear them for effect. Wearing high-heeled shoes makes a *huge* difference in how you feel about yourself. You are making a statement. If you are not quite confident enough to go for it just yet, believe me, by the end of the program you will be stepping out in those stilettos—if not actually, at least metaphorically.

Feeling good works to focus your attention elsewhere than the need for food to make you feel better.

## BOREDOM

Boredom is a hazard when you are trying to change patterns of behavior, especially when you are trying to lose weight. This is because there is, for many of us, a default setting to

| Time Needed to Complete Action |  | 1 hour |
| --- | --- | --- |

**ACTION**

Time to sort out your shoes.

If you keep your shoes in a place where you can't easily get to them, you will consistently wear the ones that are nearest to hand—whether or not they are the best ones for you.

Put aside half an hour or an hour of your time and pull out all your shoes. Lay them out on the floor in color order.

Ask yourself which of these you really want as part of the new you.

Anything tatty and old, throw away—immediately.

Out of the rest, put only the ones you love back into your wardrobe.

Put the rest in a black bag. Do not throw them away yet—you will go back to them in the final sorting exercise.

Put your loveliest, sexiest pair of shoes on—and notice how you feel. If you don't have a pair, or they are outdated or shabby—make time to go shoe shopping—if only to try them on.

our thought processes. When we are between jobs, or can't think of what to do next, especially when we don't *want* to do the next job, our unconscious mind makes a direct suggestion to us. Eat something. It will fill the gap. Put the kettle on and make a cup of tea. Have a cookie with it, or some toast. This behavior develops out of giving ourselves a treat or reward when we have completed something. It then develops into a perfect procrastination technique when we don't want to do the next job.

Rather than my telling you to distract yourself from the boredom by just getting on with the next job (which will only work for a very small percentage of people anyway—and then only for a short while), I have already given you some suggestions in CD track one. Within those suggestions I worked on a number of elements to your boredom. First, *why* is it that you feel bored? Second, why do you use food to alleviate the boredom? I did this to double your chances of breaking this particular habit, on the one hand by breaking the initial trigger—your reason for getting bored—and on the other by breaking down your connection with food as a replacement for action. As with the other suggestions, there is no need to think about them. If they apply to you, you will be able to take them on board. You may find that the reasons behind your overeating have absolutely *nothing* to do with craving food, but will have an entirely different origin.

You can find out if boredom eating is a problem for you by doing this very short exercise.

| Time Needed to Complete Action |  | 10 minutes |
|---|---|---|

**ACTION**

Have a pad and paper handy and sit or lie down with your eyes closed.

Imagine yourself going through a typical day, starting from the moment you wake. As you do, I want you to fast-forward to your habitual snack breaks. Open your eyes and make a note of them, including the time, place, and what it was you ate.

Next, close your eyes again, and just allow yourself to feel bored. Think of all the jobs that you don't want to get on with, any irritating bits to your day, and situations or even people who bore you. Now I want you to notice the sensations in your body. Are you starting to feel empty? If you have identified jobs, people, or situations that bore you, write them down on your pad.

If as a result of that short exercise you feel like reaching for the cookie jar—you have achieved a result. You have now identified a major trigger for overeating. You will now connect with the suggestions from the CD designed to help you overcome this. As I have mentioned before, one of the nicest things about the whole process of hypnotherapy is that once you have identified the problem consciously, you can use the hypnosis to get to work on your unconscious. There is no further need for you to do anything at all. You will, however, notice that as the weeks go by, your connection to boredom eating will diminish and eventually fade altogether. Around a month after completing this program, you will be able to look at your list of habitual snack breaks and notice the changes that you have made. It is important that you are hardly aware of the changes as they are happening, as you are less likely to try to sabotage them if the new patterns and habits are not dramatic, but gradual. When you add up all of the small changes that you will have made by the end of the program, you will be left with a whole new outlook—not only on your weight and your body, but also on what you are capable of achieving in your life.

If you did not come up with anything in the exercise, then the unconscious part of your mind will, as a result, be able to become more focused on your specific reasons for overeating. For every reason you eliminate you get closer to finding the key to your weight problem. The exercises in this book are designed to help you do just this. The intention is to get you to a point where you are aware of the moods, triggers, and patterns that form your current relationship with food. Then your ability to take on board the relevant hypnotherapy suggestions and retrain yourself will happen naturally.

The suggestions in the hypnosis will help you remain in

control of your eating and exercise patterns. This will be relevant for everyone who listens to the CD. You will unconsciously develop new habits—ones that can change and develop to accommodate your life and any changes that occur. Ensuring that you change your habits is one thing—making sure that you have sufficient strength and flexibility to accommodate change without slipping back into old patterns is another. I will cover this in a later section of the book.

## SETTING YOURSELF UP FOR A GOOD DAY

There are some days when we don't feel like getting out of bed. We lie there, saying to ourselves, *"Just five more minutes, then I will get up . . ."* and the more we say it, the more we convince ourselves what a good idea it is to lie there. It rarely is just five minutes. Whether we're hitting the snooze button on our alarm clocks or drifting in and out of sleep, if we don't get up straightaway that five minutes can easily turn into half an hour or even an hour. When we do wake, it is often with a jolt and a thumping heart as we realize we're going to be late. Feeling stressed, we either rush breakfast or, more commonly, skip it altogether and grab something high-calorie on the way to work and eat it in a hurry. The net result is that without our intending it, that "extra five minutes in bed" has put our eating habits out of sync for the rest of the day.

When you first become aware of your surroundings in the morning, you are not fully awake, but in what's called the hypnopompic state. Your body may feel heavy, as if it is still asleep. Your mind, however, is clear, and you are highly suggestible. The few moments when you wake are vital to how you set yourself up for the rest of the day. When you get up as soon as you wake up, rather than drifting off again, you feel much more refreshed. You also wake much more relaxed because not only do you now have time to do all the things that you need to do in the morning but you also *feel* that you have more time. Also you are not as stressed as you would be if you waited for your "startle" response to kick in. If you wake stressed, *your body wakes hungry*. Your system reacts to the stress by craving food—often sweet, high-calorie food.

Let's talk about the future. There is an old saying, "What you see is what you get." Really it should be "What you *believe* will happen is what you will get." Each and every one of us creates our own version of the present by predicting our future. Think about it. Have you ever woken up in the morning, looked through the window, seen that it is raining outside, and said to yourself: "Today is going to be a rotten day"? And guess what happens? You were right. It is called a self-fulfilling prophecy. The day was perfectly okay until you *decided* how you were going to *react* to events. This process happens to us each and every day of our lives. Making changes happen and

making them stick around long enough to become unconscious habits and responses will often start with a conscious
decision about how we are going to react to the world from
the moment we wake.

From now on you are going to use those precious moments
first thing in the morning to set yourself up for a *good* day. I
know that it will feel clumsy at first, but when you start doing
this and begin to see the effect of these new, positive suggestions in the day, which then go on to become reality, you will
soon start to make these suggestions automatically—without
even thinking about them. You really will start to notice the difference in how your day begins and develops. This is the true
power of autosuggestion—and from the point in time when
you listen to the third CD track, you will program yourself for
success each and every day before you are even fully awake
and able to talk yourself out of success.

In CD track three, which is at the start of Chapter 9, I suggest to you that when you wake, you will lie in bed for a few
minutes, and during that time you will give yourself three
positive suggestions to set you up nicely for the day. It is better to allow your unconscious mind to come up with the suggestions at the time than to try to plan them the night before.
You might suggest that *"I will have a lot of energy today,"* and
that *"I will stay calm and focused no matter what is going on
around me,"* and one, just one, suggestion relating to eating

habits or exercise, such as, *"Today I will have a walk at lunchtime."* You can repeat these suggestions to yourself for a minute or two, and at the same time drink a glass of water as you wake. It is really important that you get into the habit of drinking a large glass of water before you go to sleep, and another when you wake. We can get very dehydrated when sleeping, and can then mistake thirst for hunger.

When you build these small—and on their own insignificant—changes into your life, you will quickly notice the big changes that start to happen. I will build these suggestions into the hypnosis in such a way that you will not even be aware when you start acting on them.

Setting your "attitude alarm" in the morning has a *huge* impact on how you react to the day. If you are technologically savvy, you can vary this by recording a suggestion onto your PDA, MP3, or phone, and set the alarm so that this suggestion wakes you up. Incredible as it sounds, if the first voice you hear is one that is encouraging you, that is the attitude that you will carry with you for the rest of the day. If you don't like your own voice, ask someone else (whom you like and respect) to record it for you. I will often discourage people from waking to the radio simply because you have no control over what song will be playing when the alarm goes off. If you wake to a dirge, or even an upbeat song with sad associations, you can feel miserable for the rest of the day—even though

| Time Needed to Complete Action |  | 30 minutes |
|---|---|---|

List some positive suggestions that you would like to give yourself on waking.

*Examples:*

*Today is going to be a good day.*

*Today I will feel relaxed about (put any event that you may have been dreading, e.g., meeting the boss, taking my driving test).*

*I will enjoy myself today.*

*Today I will be motivated and (put any task here, e.g., Go for a ten-minute walk/write three pages on my book).*

Record your message.

It isn't ideal but if you really have no means of recording the suggestion electronically, put it down on paper and leave it where you will see it first thing in the morning.

you may not be aware of what triggered it. Do not underestimate the impact of the first things that you think and register with your senses when you wake.

Once you have given yourself the positive suggestions, throw off the covers and get out of bed. Staying there only makes it harder—as does using the snooze button.

When you are up, have a good stretch and a yawn. Exaggerate it. I usually find that this makes me laugh—the thought of how I must look with my mouth thrown wide open and my limbs stretched as long as possible. Once you have stretched out, you are then fully wide awake and can get on with the day. You will need to do this deliberately for the first couple of weeks, and then you will notice that it starts to become automatic. When you start the day right, with a positive suggestion and a good, old-fashioned stretch, you are on the right track for a good day. When I need an extra lift, I play one of the tracks that I have transferred onto my iPod just for this purpose while I am getting showered, "The Bear Necessities" from the *Jungle Book*—it works for me!

As with the other suggestions in this book, I have supplemented them in the hypnosis tracks.

# LIVING IN THE PRESENT

IN THIS CHAPTER I BRING TOGETHER THE SECOND SECTION of the program, in which you have worked on your present, with some of the other factors that have affected your weight in the here and now. This chapter ends with you listening to the CD track *Present,* on which all the knowledge is sent back to your unconscious where new behaviors will be triggered.

But first I will walk you through what is going to be suggested in the second track, and also *how* these suggestions will make a difference to you. Most people respond to suggestions more readily when they know what the suggestions are designed to do. That way, you can decide consciously whether you think these are the type of suggestions that relate to you specifically. Oddly enough, when we have an opportunity to evaluate suggestions before someone makes them to us, we sometimes change our mind about whether to act on them. We feel that we have more control, and then can decide if we want to do something or not. One of the most ironic misconceptions about hypnosis is that somehow, someone is going to make suggestions to you without your even realizing it, and that you will then carry them out without any free will. If anything, clinical hypnosis is the reverse. You *become more aware of suggestions* and you then *become more selective about what you choose to do.* The end result of the hypnotherapy is that you are able to make the type of suggestions to yourself that will work for you. You will no longer be susceptible to the negative self-talk that used to affect the way you felt about yourself and influenced your eating habits.

Once you develop the habit of selecting suggestions for yourself, it will play a major role in helping you to decide, both consciously and unconsciously, which ones you take on board. Remember that with all of the suggestions in this book and on the CD, you will always control the ones you ultimately choose for the changes you need in your life. Every day we are bombarded with suggestions—and we already pay attention only to those we feel have some relevance to us. The difference with the suggestions in this program is that they are designed to consistently break down negative influences, and to put in place self-selected suggestions that will work.

Let me give you an example of one way you may have succumbed to suggestion. It is a fair bet that you have browsed through a magazine at some point and found your attention drawn to the front cover of one that said something like "Drop a dress size in one week" or "A bikini body in three days." So you buy the magazine—and when you go to the article to read it, you see nothing there that you didn't know already. Now, you are a rational grown-up, so why did you fall for it—*again?* You bought the magazine not because you really believed that there was some magic formula in there for you, but because of your *mood*—and it is that mood-dependent vulnerability that I am going to help you eliminate once and for all with this program.

Once you can become aware of your mood triggers you will start to notice the automatic behaviors that you developed in response to those moods. In the second CD track I will lead you through a sequence of suggestions to help you do just that. The ability to respond differently to the moods, or to divert them altogether if they are no longer appropriate to you, will follow in the three weeks after listening to this track.

The second session is designed to help you recognize and deal with patterns of thought, behavior, and emotion. The impact of becoming aware of what *you can change* is significant. The hypnosis track will help you in two specific ways. First, it will give direct suggestions to help you pay attention to the things that you can control rather than those that you feel that you can't change. This is a significant shift—because when this happens, you start to feel more able to let go of the things that you cannot control.

In the second track, I also look at the ways in which you act, think, and feel as a person with a weight problem. These are the things that currently bind you and keep you from recognizing how easy it is for you to start making the changes you can make to become a different version of yourself.

## PLUS ONE EQUALS MISERY; MINUS ONE EQUALS HAPPINESS

This program is not abstract theory. I have worked successfully with many people over the years on the issues of self-image and weight. What I haven't mentioned before is the reason why I don't just feel that it works, but I *know*. I was a chunky kid and a heavy teenager. In fact, for the first thirty years of my life I had a very unhappy relationship with my body. I would weigh myself daily, and what I saw on the scales told me whether I was going to have a good day or a bad day. If I was the same weight as the day before, I knew that I would have an average sort of day. If, heaven forbid, I had put on a couple of ounces, then I was going to be miserable. If I had lost weight, I knew it was going to be a *good* day.

Those bathroom scales became more than an indicator of my weight—they became my fortune-teller. It didn't matter how I lost the weight: whether it was because I had been ill, or even because I had deliberately thrown up because I had binged, the net result was the same. I had lost weight, so I was happy, and that was all there was to it. My weight was my obsession—and I knew that I was not alone. I started to recognize others who had similar obsessions. They were the women whom, if you asked them, "Have you lost weight?" would beam happily and say "Not really—well, maybe a couple of pounds" and would stay happy for the rest of the day, just because of what I had said to them. I also knew this mood swing would occur *regardless* of whether they had actually lost any weight, and was simply because they *felt better about themselves.*

There was one single equation in my mind, and that was: Slim = Happy, popular, successful. On the other hand, the opposite equation was just as real: Fat = Unhappy, unpopular, and unsuccessful. When I did an impartial assessment of my weight and my success in other areas of life (exams, jobs, partnerships), I could trace a direct correlation between feeling good about myself and losing weight—but I always lost the weight *after* I felt good about myself in other areas of my life—not before. The weight loss was a response, not a trigger to my success. Feeling good about yourself is the key to long-term change—not the numbers that you see on a scale. By the end of this program you will not only recognize this in practical terms, but you will also make an emotional connection with this statement—one that will help and guide you through the many and varied stages of your life from now on.

## MOOD CONTROL USING HYPNOSIS

Until you have gotten yourself fully under conscious control, you can use the mood-control suggestions that you will find in track two of the CD. In this track, I have three different sets of suggestions to help you:

1. Change your mood before it gets hold of you and unwanted behavior kicks in.
2. Divert it before it becomes damaging.
3. Stop it if it is still strong enough to get an initial hold on you.

These three tactics, which either halt, help you cope with, or interrupt your mood swing, will give you a belt-and-suspenders approach to getting control over your mood. If one does not work, then another will help you, and you have an extra one left over if all else fails.

Controlling the moods that used to trigger the habitual patterns in relation to body image and eating can be the hardest habits to break. Stopping smoking is easier, as you can at least tell when you have succeeded—you either smoke or you don't. However, when it comes to having control over our feelings it is a sliding scale, so it is harder to tell when we are winning. The hypnosis will help you here, too, getting you to focus on the areas of your life over which you do have control, and therefore creating new habits of attention to the positives, rather than dwelling on failures as you probably have done up until now.

## AN UNEVEN PLAYING FIELD

There are reasons why some of us are predisposed to be bigger than others. There are other reasons to do with lifestyle that we can control, and by the end of the program you will have the necessary tools to manage your lifestyle. To truly take control of your weight and your body image means to learn to accept certain aspects of yourself that cannot be altered. In accepting them, you remove the associated stress.

There is a whole section on track two of the CD that is designed to help you to do just this.

It is, however, worth me spelling out to you the reasons why you *may* have found it so much harder than other people to lose weight. I do this for one reason alone, so that you can realize that—if these reasons apply to you—then, yes, it was harder for you. That is why you will come out of this process so much stronger than before—because you will not only have taken control of your weight and your body image, but you will also know yourself well enough to stop fooling yourself into thinking that you cannot change things. You can and you will because you will *focus on the things that you can change, and let go of those that you cannot.*

You may also discover that you don't actually have a predisposition for weight gain and that you are in a better position to change your weight and your body image than you imagined.

One reason you may find it hard to lose weight may be due to what happened to you before you were born. It appears that there is some interuterine programming that relates specifically to our relationships with food. If you are born to an obese mother, especially one who developed diabetes while pregnant, you are much more likely to go on to develop obesity in later life. Conversely, babies born of mothers who were subjected to famine conditions (studies on this subject were done on postwar babies in Holland) are statistically more likely to go on to develop obesity when they have unlimited access to food.

Now, what happened to us before we were born is something that we cannot alter. However, by acknowledging that it may be a factor, you can take steps to watch your food intake—just as you would take steps to wear sunblock if you inherited fair skin.

*Just by the act of reading this book you are already beginning to take responsibility.*

For the majority of us, however, our mothers were neither obese nor starving—and so the concept of maladaptive pre-birth programming causing you to be fat applies only to a small percentage of the population.

On the subject of pregnancy, you might be interested in a pattern I have observed over many years of one-to-one practice. I have treated countless women who were trying to get pregnant. Often these women are fit and food conscious, statistically a little older than the average for a first pregnancy, but in most instances there can be found no specific physical reason for their infertility. I noticed that every one of them had been on a diet at some time in their lives. Each one shared an unacknowledged fear of "getting fat" in pregnancy, and every one of them was slightly underweight. A big part of the psychological work I did with them was to get their body image under control and allow them to feel okay about their changing shape during pregnancy. Our unconscious mind has a wonderful way of protecting us from change if it feels that we are in danger in any way. For those women whose self-esteem was connected to a fixed notion of body image, it was not surprising that they had problems getting pregnant—or as their unconscious was framing it, getting fat. Once we had worked on the body image, I then encouraged them to eat a little more in preparation for pregnancy. This put them into the normal weight range and—hey presto—pregnant.

I mention this as it is a fact that in terms of our basic physiology we are geared up to respond in very primitive ways when we perceive danger around us. Stress equals danger; danger equals "This is not a good time to have a baby." Women have an extraordinarily strong connection with the unconscious part of the mind designed to protect us. When this connection goes out of whack we lose control of certain behaviors and responses, and lose a real sense of our physical selves. *However, by the end of the program you will be listening to yourself in a way that is designed to protect you—a way that will help you fully understand the messages from this part of yourself.*

## ACCEPT WHAT YOU CANNOT CHANGE—
## CHANGE EVERYTHING ELSE

For the majority of us, there is very little we cannot modify—from what we eat to how much activity is in our lives. However, part of taking control of our feelings about our bodies and our weight includes recognizing that there are things we cannot change. This frees up the mind to concentrate on the things we can.

Most of us will have gotten into the habit of looking for excuses for our weight gain, and the more we read that gives us a "reason" (or excuse) for why we are overweight, the more likely we are to do nothing active to change it. Changing things means taking responsibility as well as control, and can be a really scary thought if you lack confidence. That is why, all the way through the hypnosis tracks, you will find suggestions on creating confident states, on creating emotional flexibility, and on being proud of your achievements. Confidence is the bedrock for long-term change. For the majority of us, *feeling confident* is not an issue of how much we weigh, but of self-esteem. We have habitually equated weight with how we feel about ourselves. *Now is the time to break that habit once and for all.*

## FINDING A PARTNER LIKE YOU

Why is it that when some women get into long-term relationships with a partner they put on weight, and it stays there? It has a little to do with like finding like, a little to do with biochemistry, and a lot to do with habits and the ways in which most women change their behavior to fit into their new partner's lifestyle—more specifically, the lifestyle that they believe will define them as a couple. Couples (especially in the first stages of living together) spend a lot of time on the sofa or in activities that allow them to talk and relax in each other's company. If the relationship is highly charged sexually—great. Otherwise there is often very little exercise going on.

Add to this the fact that more takeout meals will be bought because, unless one or both partners love cooking, neither partner will want to immediately take on the role of chef. Taking on the role of chef is the next step into domesticity, and so some couples unconsciously avoid it. Also when couples first live together, cooking is not the first thing on their minds. This in itself is not a problem, unless it goes on for a few weeks and settles into a habit of "If it is Friday, we have takeout curry." When takeout meals become a habit rather than something you think about, you soon find that you stop thinking about it as food and your ability to assess how much you are eating, and how fattening the food is will soon be forgotten. The other problem with takeout food is that you don't really notice how much more you are eating—that is, until you start to notice that your clothes are getting a bit tight. The trouble is, by now you are already in a habit, and in the early stages of a relationship you are not really very motivated to start doing things differently.

Takeout should be seen as a treat—not a habit. Don't cut it out altogether if you really enjoy it—but here is a tip to make you think twice. When you next get a takeout meal, before you eat it—weigh it. It will absolutely horrify you. The last time I ordered a set meal for two from my local Chinese restaurant, I put it on the bathroom scale. It came in at a stunning seven pounds three ounces—and I was about to eat half of that. Since then I have stopped ordering the set meals, as I now realize that there is simply too much food there. When I do order, I order *enough*. Takeout is fine, but order sensibly—and make it a treat rather than a habit. Better still—go out. You will end up having a better evening all around, and the more effort you have to make, the more you will enjoy yourself.

There is another reason why some women can get bigger when they move into a stable relationship, and that is that they decide to use the contraceptive pill. Just as when you stop smoking, it is not inevitable that you will put on weight, but it is something to be aware of. I have created some catch-all suggestions in track two to make sure that you do not create bad habits from your excuses, and to make you more conscious of the food decisions you make from now on.

## A CHILD'S MIND IN AN ADULT'S BODY

We cannot trace every pattern and habit back to our childhood, but it is still true that the majority of our attitudes, behaviors, and responses have their roots there. In many instances where appropriate, we grow out of them as we change and develop into adults. But other patterns of behavior hang around us, an unwanted and unnecessary reminder of childhood.

Understanding why you have a problem is the beginning of change, not the end. This is where the hypnotherapeutic component of this program really comes into its own. It allows you to go into your own mental space, identify the relevant childhood "hangovers," and overwrite them with healthy, appropriate adult reactions. This is not about blaming anyone for what happened to you as a child. This is about taking responsibility for your health and happiness as an adult. Once you have let go of certain feelings, you will more easily be able to let go of the behaviors associated with those

## CASE | HISTORY

**A CHILD'S MIND IN AN ADULT'S BODY**

Sally found that whenever she got sad she reached for chocolate cookies. It didn't matter what it was that made her sad, even if she was watching a commercial for the ASPCA on TV. She found herself automatically reaching for the chocolate cookies, and then felt even worse because she didn't actually want them. I worked with Sally using hypnosis to help her feel better about herself generally, and become aware of what it was from her own personal history that meant that she felt this need to express her sadness. Sally remembered that when she was young and her mother was taken into the hospital, she was cared for by her grandmother. Her grandmother gave her chocolate cookies—something that wasn't allowed at home. She had unconsciously associated the sadness of her mother's illness with eating chocolate cookies. When she became aware of this, she took control of the eating habit, realizing it was just a throwback from her past and not something relevant to her present. She still occasionally ate them—but not in response to the mood that used to trigger such behavior. Sally lost twenty-eight pounds in six months as a result of this change alone.

feelings. As with many of the concepts in this program, you do not need to think too much about whether they relate to

## HYPNOSIS | SESSION 2

**THE PRESENT**

| Time Needed to Complete Action |  | 20 minutes |

### ACTION

Track two: *Present*

Go to the toilet if you need to.

Turn off your phone and minimize other possible distractions.

Choose a time and find a place where you can be undisturbed. You can sit down or lie down, as long as you are comfortable. Do not cross your arms or legs; allow them to relax.

If you wear glasses, take them off.

Close your eyes.

Now listen to the second track on the CD, called *Present*.

When the track is over, sit or lie still for a few moments to make sure you are fully reoriented.

Remember: if anything happens that requires your attention while you are listening to the CD, you will become fully alert and able to respond.

If you want to write down anything that you thought or felt as part of listening to the hypnosis track, do so now. You can review it again later before continuing with the program.

I suggest that once you have listened to the hypnosis track, you read no further today. You can pick it up again tomorrow.

you or not—the hypnosis tracks will help you work this out as you work through the relevant suggestions. The events of our formative years are critical in forming our framework for adult life in many ways. Our memories, however, play tricks on us. Not everything we think we remember is accurate— nor will all the memories that we *think* are relevant actually turn out to be so.

This is why, in the next hypnosis track, I concentrate on the effects of memory. Memories in themselves cannot be altered, but the ways in which we feel about them—and, more significantly, respond to them—*can* be changed. Among the hypnosis suggestions in track two, you will be aware of one that concentrates on memory and how you relate to your past. At no point will you be asked to recall past events, nor will you spontaneously recall anything that you are not able to deal with. The hypnosis suggestions are delivered to you in such a way that you will always control them, and be safe with them. Remember this and you will be fine. This track is a form of mental housekeeping, designed to help you get rid of connections that are no longer useful or valid, and to access and look forward to creating strong, positive memories.

The CD track also contains suggestions for your confidence—*to enable you to be more in control every day.*

<br>

C
H
A
P
T
E
R

·

7

# CHANGE WHAT YOU CAN CHANGE, ACCEPT WHAT YOU CAN'T

WITH THIS CHAPTER, WE MOVE INTO THE FINAL SECTION of the program. You have listened to two hypnosis CD tracks so far, *Past* and *Present*. This final section is about the future. It's time to get serious about change and make real progress. The two hypnosis sessions that you have completed so far have now set you up to start making these changes without thinking too much about what you are doing. In this chapter we concentrate on removing temptation, creating a space for the new you, and recognizing the new patterns of behavior that need to happen to make these changes consistent and permanent. I have also included a few simple food tips and recipes to keep you on track.

This chapter is also about clearing the decks in order to receive the new you, and about making sure that you will not be tempted into the old, negative ways of behaving. This new you will be free from mood swings and will no longer hide behind baggy clothes or comfort eating. Hypnosis helps to break those kinds of negative patterns once and for all.

## DETOX

I bet you were wondering how long it would be before you saw the word *detox*, right? Well, here is the news. Don't do it. Drinking lemon juice for a week, or cabbage soup, or vegetable smoothies . . . stop right there! You can take it from me as a former detox junkie that as a route to long-term change and contentment with your body, detoxes just don't work.

I have done them all (or most of them) at one time or another. I have traveled the world of detox spas, from India to Austria, and have found them to be populated in general by gaunt and anemic evangelists and a smattering of normal people suffering from the effects of overwork, overeating, and lack of sleep. There is no question that when I left the spa doors and returned home (armed with my prison-ration bread to teach me to chew properly, and my list of food and obscure shops where I could continue with my supply of "healthy eating" products) I did feel better, and my vital signs reflected this. The *real* benefit of these detoxes, however, is that you are away from your normal day-to-day stressors, including pollution, work, and noise. It's not surprising that you're going to feel better as a result. But if you ask medical practitioners for their opinion on the whole concept of detoxing from food, as I did when researching this book, most will agree that to detox is pointless at best, and potentially damaging to the digestive system at worst. There are, certainly, exceptions to the rule if you have a genuine intolerance to specific foods, but these are exceptions. *Most* people do not need to detoxify their bodies. Their lifestyles, yes; their bodies, no.

## A glass of hot water with lemon juice and honey

A doctor friend of mine recommended that if I wanted to be able to pay attention to my body's food requirements, it would be very useful to start the day with a sharp flavor to wake up the taste buds. I now start my day with a large glass of hot water with lemon juice and honey. It took a bit of getting used to at first, being a little too healthy for my usual tastes, and a bit too close to a detox, but I gave it a go. Now it is essential to starting my day properly.

There are many differing benefits claimed for this mixture. None of them as far as I am aware have much research behind them. Claims for this mixture range from promoting weight loss by increasing urination and alkalinity to promoting a detoxifying effect to the calming and destressing capabilities of the honey content. For me it is a very good way to wake up, as it gives me my sweet "fix" for the day in a way that also clears my palette. I find that after drinking it I can decide more easily whether I am hungry for sweet or savory content in my first meal of the day. This prevents the confusing situation of finding yourself having eaten your breakfast, knowing that you *should* be full, but still craving something else. When you listen to your body and move away from an automatic breakfast you will end this pattern. And as we've seen, by drinking a large glass of water before a meal you are also less likely to confuse thirst and hunger—which is a common problem for many people.

As with many of the other suggestions in this program, some of you will really respond to this, and if it is appropriate for you, you will take on board the suggestions by picking up on the relevant sections in the final CD track.

## TROMPE L'OEIL (AND YOUR OTHER SENSES)

Trompe l'oeil is a term used in art to describe a way of painting designed to alter your perception, and for me it is a useful term when it comes to food and your perception of what you eat. To really change your eating habits for life you need to initially trick more than your eyes. You need to trick all of your senses into being satisfied. If you can engage all of your senses with the food you are about to eat, then you are more than halfway to changing your mind-set about what you eat and how full(filled) you are going to feel afterward.

Remember here that you have more than one sense to satisfy—your eyes, your ears, your touch, and your smell. Taste is the last of the senses to satisfy. The others all help prepare your body to enjoy and digest your food properly. Let me give you an example. If you take a tomato from the fridge, and eat it there and then, you know it will taste of nothing much at all. The cold sensation can be quite unpleasant (especially if you have sensitive teeth) and the texture feels bland on your palette. When you bite into it, it tastes of almost nothing, so you may put salt or mayonnaise on it to pep it up when actually there is a much better and easier way of getting flavor into it.

Have you noticed that holiday food always tastes better, no matter how simple it is? A plate of tomatoes with cheese, olive oil, and basil eaten in a simple trattoria can be incredibly satisfying. Why do you think that is? First, it is because you are feeling relaxed, and therefore your digestion is relaxed too. I have already talked about the importance of this earlier in the book, and there are many suggestions in the CD tracks to help you with this. The other factor here is that food should not be eaten cold, straight from the fridge—ever. We have become so obsessed with the idea that most of our food needs to be kept chilled that we stick it all in the fridge and expect it to give up all its flavors automatically when we then pull it out. My kitchen smells. You read it here first. My kitchen smells of tomatoes and herbs and cheese, of bread and fruit. It smells of food and cooking. It seems as if we have become afraid of our sense of smell—as if everything has to be smell-free to be hygienic. By putting everything in the fridge we seem to have developed a pattern that means that we don't allow our senses to become prepared to eat. Our bodies require time and stimulation to prepare themselves before we put something in our mouths. Without time and stimulation, we do not have the right gustatory juices ready to digest the food, and will very quickly get bloated, and indigestion will follow.

Food also tastes better on your holiday because you are having a break from the stress of your normal life. If you like, you are detoxing from stress and therefore able to digest food in a more healthy way. You will also have been feeding your other senses during your holiday. Looking at different scenery, smelling different smells, hearing different languages—these all involve your senses. Food then becomes one of many nice experiences. It is important for you to enjoy your mealtimes. Make them about more than just the food. Put some music on, set the table. Make it into a special event whenever you can. You will be surprised at how much difference this makes. Take your time, and enjoy food as part of life. It is not something to suffer from or avoid. Embrace it—you will quickly find that you awaken other appetites as well.

So, here is the key. Prepare yourself and your food, and set the scene *properly* for eating. I know what you are thinking: "What about work—there is often little or no chance of preparing food properly. It's a quick sandwich at the desk if I'm lucky." Remember, we all have choices and there will be times when it is impossible to do anything except grab food and eat it at your desk. But please don't use this time to read a women's magazine or a health publication. If you must read while you're eating, pick up a home-improvement magazine or a book, or a holiday brochure instead. I know it sounds obvious, but if you are looking at pictures of skinny women while you are eating your unsatisfying sandwich on the run you will be reinforcing images of negative stereotypes and you will end up feeling not only that you have not enjoyed your food but also that any feeling of fullness is revolting—you will *feel fat.* Even though you have only had a small amount of food, looking at those skinny women sends your brain mixed messages—

so stop it right now. This is a simple enough action—and it will help your brain to respond appropriately to the food that you *are* eating.

And finally, a quick question: when did you last consider the size of your plate in relation to the size of your stomach? Use smaller plates. You will soon notice how much more quickly you feel full when you have a loaded small plate, rather than a large plate looking sparse—or worse still, filling up your large plate because it doesn't look like enough food. You might be interested to know that plate size has increased by 30 percent in the last fifteen years—but your stomach hasn't.

## ALCOHOL

If you do not drink alcohol, you needn't read this section. If, however, you do drink alcohol, consider this: alcohol doesn't only add empty calories of its own, but under its influence you are more likely to overeat, and once you are feeling the hangover, you are even more likely to reach for food as a comfort to distract you from how unwell you feel. Do not underestimate the massive benefits in terms of weight loss and general health and well-being that stem from taking a break from booze.

There is only one place in the program where I suggest that you fast—and here it is. By cutting out alcohol completely for three weeks you will notice a rapid change in how you feel and look. Significantly, you will lose weight without changing your eating habits.

Abstaining from alcohol is the only type of detox worth doing because it gives your liver time to recover. Without question you will *feel better, healthier, and more energetic* as a result. For many of us with our busy modern lifestyles, I recognize that this can seem like the hardest detox, as drinking alcohol can become so much a part of our lives—and more significantly—our relaxation time. The fact is that alcohol is a muscle relaxant, and drinking is a quick and easy way of slipping out of our daily routine and into a more comfortable feeling. The major problem with this is that it can quickly shift into becoming a habit—especially if you are not happy.

It is a commonly held belief in many parts of the world that one *needs* alcohol to have a good time. It is simply not true. Think about it. When you were much younger, before you ever drank alcohol, you were perfectly capable of having fun—and if you really think about it, you should be able to re-member plenty of times when you have had a good time with-out alcohol being in the mix. If you can't recall having a good time without alcohol, or if the mere thought of going without it for three weeks makes you break out in a cold sweat—then you may have a genuine drinking problem. If you have a genuine concern about being dependent on alcohol, then do consult your GP.

If you drink alcohol, reducing your intake is the quickest and easiest way of losing weight. For the next three weeks I want you to go about your daily life, do all the things you would normally do, but without alcohol. You will quickly find that other people do not care or, in most instances, even notice that you are not drinking. We persuade ourselves that if we don't have a drink when we are out with our friends, *"just to be sociable"* then they will notice—but there is a contradiction. When people are drinking they become less aware of other people's behavior. Not only that, but you will notice theirs more. When you have three weeks without alcohol you will have given your liver time to recover. Your metabolism will regulate more effectively, and you will sleep better. You will also be able to get a clearer picture of any areas of your life that are problems for you—something that drinking may have masked. Once the fast is over, you will find that any habitual connection with drinking alcohol will be eliminated, and you will be able to be more selective about when and how much you do drink—finding that you prefer the feeling of being in control to being out of it. I like a drink— occasionally. I drink to celebrate, and for that reason will stick to champagne. It is lower in calories but more expensive, so I have to think twice before buying it—and when I do drink it, I will be in a happy mood. We all know that alcohol amplifies the mood you are in when you drink it—so I enhance my mood when it is a good one. Again, having a three-week fast from alcohol will enable you to recognize much more clearly those things that stress you about your life. In doing so, you will be well on the way to taking control of them as you continue with this program.

Track three of the CD contains all the suggestions you will need to help you with the alcohol fast and to notice the benefits as you are doing it. Some people decide, as a result of the fast, to repeat it whenever they are feeling sluggish or bloated. Others fast after a holiday or when they have eaten and drunk more than they usually would. It is always there for you—do not underestimate the power of it.

A tip to help you during this fast is to change the glass from which you drink your chosen alternatives. Don't use a tumbler; use a wineglass or, better still, a champagne flute. When you are holding a wineglass, even if the contents are not wine, a psychological shift takes place. This allows you to fool your brain long enough to get over the feeling that you might be missing out on something by not drinking. Your mental associations of alcohol are also linked to the actions that you make when drinking—so holding the stem or bowl of a wineglass instead of a boring old tumbler will allow you to hold on to the pleasant associations of drinking alcohol—without the ill effects the next morning. It can also fool others. Remember, most people do not pay attention to what (or how much) other people are drinking, but if it bothers you that other people might wonder why you are not drinking alcohol, then a wineglass will ensure that *they will not notice at all*. It also helps to have a jug of water and a nonalcoholic alternative on the table when you are having dinner parties.

What you drink instead is entirely up to you. If you want to fool other people (and yourself) that you are drinking alcohol, you can mix anything with tonic water or sparkling water. Some of my favorite mixers are cranberry, elderflower, and clear apple juice. Sparkling water with a splash of lime juice in a champagne glass is my ideal drink of choice when going alcohol free. If you like something with a bit of bite, there are alcohol-free wines and beers around (some of them are surprisingly good). Do remember that some of the off-the-shelf drinks can be packed full of sugar—so read the label carefully.

## DRUGS

In addition to everything else we ingest, some of us also take prescription medication. Have you ever considered whether your medication is causing you to put on weight? Studies on medication types such as euroleptics, anticonvulsants, antihypertensives, beta-blockers, diabetes medication, and the contraceptive pill have shown potential side effects of weight gain in the individual taking the medication over a two-year period ranging from two and a half to eleven pounds (1.2 to 5 kg). Before you start blaming your medication for weight gain, however, take a step back from the statistics for a moment. What is often not accounted for in studies is the changes in metabolism caused by the condition that these medications are designed to treat. Nor is there always reliable, detailed data on the diet and lifestyles of those participating in the studies. Weight gain with medication is *not* inevitable. If you have a condition that means that you need to take medication, you may already have been told that you need to make improvements to your diet and lifestyle or that you need to lose weight as part of the treatment process.

## POLLUTION/CHEMICALS

At this time, we do not have a clear picture of the medical effects of the pollution and chemicals that are around us and in our food. Studies on mice, for example, have shown that ingesting the pesticide dieldrin caused them to double their body fat. Some chemicals contain endocrine disruptors that, in turn, influence estrogen production and increase the body's capacity to lay down its fat stores. We simply do not have enough information to make an informed choice. However, one thing is certain: eating fresh, healthy food means we have more control over what goes into our body. Some years ago I made a conscious decision to stop eating foodstuffs that contained ingredients that I couldn't spell—or identify. Effectively, this meant that I stopped eating food out of cardboard packets. "Ready-made" means that there are hidden ingredients designed solely for preservation and presentation that you simply do not need (or want) to eat. This had the added bonus of reducing my salt and sugar intake immediately, and I started to lose weight without having to try. Eating healthily is all about making choices. I order my fruit and vegetables on the Internet from a local farmers cooperative, with the added bonus of getting produce I would ordinarily not try.

## MIXING UP YOUR DIET

Think about your shopping list. How many of the items on there do you include automatically without even thinking about them? Milk, eggs, cheese, bread . . . If you want to lose weight and still be able to enjoy food—in fact, to enjoy it properly—then you need to mix it up a little. Give your taste buds variety and you are much more likely to eat less. In the last hypnosis track I made suggestions to help you shop more consciously. I suggested that you feast your eyes too, when shopping, and buy a greater variety of colors. Did you know that foods that are naturally orange in color generally have fewer calories than different-colored similar foodstuffs?

Like everybody (if they are being honest), I can get bored with salads. The temptation is to smother them in dressing to get a more pleasant taste and texture. I call it the "yum factor." You can really miss that extra flavor when you are trying to lose weight. Instead of buying ready-made sauces, you can try one of these three combinations:

- Hummus and tomato juice
- Guacamole thinned out with a little relish (the best one in the world—Henderson's Relish—comes from my hometown, Sheffield, and is suitable for vegetarians)
- Organic crunchy peanut butter and cider vinegar

Here are a couple of easy recipes included only because they, too, give you that full taste experience that is missing from low-calorie dressings.

## Caesar Salad Dressing
### LOW-CALORIE AND LOW-CHOLESTEROL VERSION

*½ cup plain low-fat yogurt*

*¼ cup each low-cal mayonnaise and lemon juice*

*2 teaspoons each chopped fresh parsley, grated Parmesan cheese, water*

*1 clove garlic, minced*

*¼ teaspoon anchovy paste (or 2 teaspoons Worcestershire sauce)*

OPTIONAL: *a few leaves of fresh oregano or basil, minced*

Put everything in a bowl and whisk until smooth. Cover it and store in fridge.

## Sesame Dressing

*1 teaspoon sesame seed*

*1 clove garlic, minced*

*2 teaspoons virgin olive oil*

*2 tablespoons vinegar*

*1 teaspoon honey*

*1 teaspoon soy sauce*

*Black pepper, to taste*

Mix it all together, store it in the fridge, and shake well before use.

## Never add salt

Adding salt to food is, for most people, a habit.

I was speaking to a headhunter recently; her job was to find chief executive officers for some of the most prominent global companies in the city. When I asked how she knew whether someone was going to be able to make it as a top executive, she told me: "If they put salt on their food before tasting it, it showed enough about their character to know that they will make decisions before they have all the facts—and they won't survive long in top-level decision making before they make a critical mistake. I simply will not put them forward to my clients if I see them do this!" Who would have thought that we give so much away by adding salt?

Reducing your salt intake has many benefits, among them lowering your blood pressure and getting rid of that bloated feeling. All in all you will find that very soon you won't miss it. Stop putting the salt out on the table and you will soon get out of the habit of automatically adding it to food. You will also feel less thirsty, which is especially beneficial for those people who sometimes mistake thirst for hunger.

## Alternative breakfasts

This is one of my favorite breakfasts in summer, and it will set you up for the rest of the day. It is sweet, healthy, and low in calories, and is a slow-release food, so it will keep you feeling full longer.

## Austrian Muesli

(MAKES ENOUGH FOR 3 TO 4 DAYS)

*4 cups oats*

*2 ounces raisins*

*1 ounce flaked almonds*

*1 small apple, diced*

*1 cup orange or apple juice*

*2 cups milk (soy or cow's)*

Mix all the dry ingredients in a bowl with the liquid and leave overnight in the fridge. The mix will seem wet but the moisture will have soaked in by the morning. Before eating, you can add fresh fruit.

I love this muesli, as you actually feel as if you are eating something naughty but nice rather than healthy. It is very filling and will last you until lunchtime—and it is great for digestion too.

# CONFIDENCE TRICKS

THIS CHAPTER IS ALL ABOUT THE DIFFERENT THINGS YOU
can do quickly and easily to feel and look better. I have called
this chapter "Confidence Tricks" because as soon as you do
something that makes you look better, you immediately *feel*
better about yourself, and your confidence is boosted—
especially when people start telling you that you look good.

So far we have concentrated on the past and the present.
From here on we will focus on the future and how you are
going to react to your body. During the three weeks following
completion of this program you are going to become aware of,

and allow yourself to recognize, the new thoughts and behaviors that are becoming part of the new you. It is also important to recognize the role of emotions and the new sensations of control that form part of your long-term change. Additionally, in this chapter I will tell you how to take control of the yo-yo of weight loss and weight gain once and for all.

This stage of the program is all about taking what you already know about yourself and what you should be doing, and creating the new you who is strong and capable of acting on this knowledge. The final section of hypnosis in Chapter 9 will fix this new self into your unconscious. Before then, I want to take you through some tricks for success and help you to "fake it until you make it."

## CONFIDENCE FROM WITHIN

Everyone has good bits—even if you can't immediately think of them. You may have nice hands or a good neck or striking eyes. Sadly, when we become obsessed with weight we forget about the areas of our body that are fine—better than fine in some cases. Ironically, just as there is one voice that you will not listen to when it comes to making suggestions for change—your own voice—so there are other voices that you are much less inclined to listen to when it comes to making objective comments on your looks. These are usually the voices of people who love you and care about you, and have said nice things to you before. You feel that they will say nice things regardless of how you actually look. This leads me neatly into an emotional no-go area—the "how do I look?" scenario.

If you want to have and maintain a good relationship with your partner, *never* ask your partner a question about your body when you are feeling insecure—and I do mean never. It puts them in an impossible situation. Men are programmed to offer solutions, and that is not what you want at all. So you ask them a question that only has one "right" answer and the partner has to guess the correct response. You can see the fear in their eyes when they hear:

*"How do I look?"*
*"What do you think of this outfit?"*
*"Do you think X is pretty?"*
*"I am not sure about this shirt, what do you think?"*

and last but not least, that old classic:

*"Does my bum look big in this?*

Men will make the mistake of trying to answer the question that you asked them—albeit in a way that they hope will please you. These are evil, wicked questions. They should be banned. You *know* why. You are not asking your partner because you want to know their opinion—you are telling them that you are feeling insecure. In most cases, what you are really saying is: *"Tell me that you love me."*

If you really feel compelled to ask your partner how you look, first *tell* your partner what you want to hear. In fact, forget asking at all, just tell them what you want to hear. Everyone will be happier. For example: *"Tell me my bum looks great in this!"* Believe me, life is so much easier that way.

The problem with these questions and the need to ask them comes not from your partner's inability to read your mind, but from the fact that you do not have enough confidence to know yourself that you look great. When you grow in confidence, you will know how good you look, and can own those feelings. You will get there—just keep working through the program. Until then, stop asking others for the reassurance you need to give yourself, as it can backfire. Better not to ask at all, and instead develop your own positive inner voice.

## POSTURE AND BREATHING

When you stand tall, there are two immediate benefits. The first is that you look slimmer. The second is that you feel better, as standing tall is the posture of confidence and control.

One thing I am blessed with is good posture. Or, to put it more accurately, I was blessed with a European mother who constantly reminded me to sit up straight, to walk with my feet pointing forward, not outward or inward, and to keep my head even and level, as if I was carrying a book on my head. She motivated me by reminding me that the taller I looked, the slimmer I seemed. When I grew up, I also noticed that this was the posture most associated with confidence, and became convinced that these two are interrelated. If you slouch, your stomach pushes out, your head slumps down, and you *look* rounder and less comfortable with yourself.

Getting your posture right takes practice, but rather than worrying about how to achieve it, the best way is to imagine you are being watched by an invisible camera and pose. You already know how you are standing when you look your best— and this is when you are confident. Practice, and use the suggestions in track three of the CD to work on your confidence (you will be prompted to listen to track three at the end of Chapter 9). Good posture will follow, as will good breathing. You can practice all you like to breathe properly, but it is only when good, deep breathing becomes an unconscious process that the benefits will really kick in. Remember—shallow breathing is associated with anxiety, so *the more confident you become, the better you will deal with situations that used to bother you* and the more your breathing will settle down into deep, even breaths, without your being conscious of making the effort. That is the real beauty of connecting with the un-conscious part of your mind—the part that knows how to best care for you. As you grow in confidence, so you grow in stature, and your posture improves. Apart from anything else, if you walk tall you *immediately* appear to have shed about seven pounds.

## MAGIC WAND

It is not called a wand for nothing—yes—you guessed it—mascara. To me, a makeup kit is pure, unadulterated magic. You can "put your face on" and greet the day feeling so much more confident and in control than without it. Given a choice, would you rather meet your ex-boyfriend with your face naked—or with some makeup on?

Putting on makeup is not only about creating yourself—a face to show the world—but it also shows that you are tak-ing time to care for yourself, that you spend time on yourself. This again comes down to the issue of self-confidence. If you get everything done but constantly look harassed and un-happy, then you are going about things backward. You come first. Remember the warning given on aircraft: "In the event of an emergency ensure that you put on your mask first be-fore helping others." Yes, I know this message is about oxygen, but the message is clear. Care for yourself *first*, or you will be in no position to care for others.

If you are not sure how to do quickie makeup, go to the cosmetics counter of a department store and tell them that you want a course in five-minute makeup. You don't have to buy the products, and you will be able to see the difference in your face immediately. By taking five minutes out to do your makeup, you will make a huge difference in how you approach your day. You are saying, *"I come first."* If you already make up your face, it is still worth visiting the cosmetic counters and letting them update you on colors and new products. Putting on makeup is about attitude. It doesn't matter how good your clothes look, if your face is not made up, you will seem unfinished. Five minutes—that is all it takes.

## SCENT-SATIONS

Different smells create different emotions. When you are changing as a person, there comes a time to update your perfume. If you have been wearing the same one for years, it is *definitely* time for a change. For one thing, your skin will have changed and by now will react to the scent differently from when you first started wearing it. Also, you and the people around you no longer smell it because it's become so familiar. So do try something new.

Putting on perfume will become an automatic response every day when you have showered and dressed. Do not leave the bedroom without it. Your scent should remind you of good times. When I buy a new perfume, I always wear it out for a special occasion *first*, and that becomes my memory associated with that scent. It means that every time I wear it, I will be reminded on an unconscious level of how good I felt the first time I wore it. It may be a very sensual, sexy evening for you and your partner, a real party night, or a walk in the countryside—whatever you choose. You will always be able to connect with those positive feelings by smelling that perfume.

## CORSETS AND BUSTIERS

Contrary to those images of progressively skinnier women that the media continues to subject us to, men like—make that *love*—women who have curves. This is not a social or a fashion trend, this is down to pure instinct. Women who have a 7:10 waist-to-hip ratio are more fertile—and men pick up on this unconsciously. This is about survival of the species.

If you look at some of the sexiest women of the last century, many of them would be considered fat by the standards of today. Look at Marilyn Monroe and Sophia Loren—there are plenty of examples out there—fabulous, sexy ladies.

If you were not blessed by nature with a small waist, create one. Wearing a structured, sexy corset (there are some wonderful styles and fabrics available now) does wonders for your outline. The best way to train yourself in it is to wear it for half an hour or so around the house and build up the time you wear it. When you can wear it easily for four hours, start wearing it out of the house. As with wearing high heels, you will notice that you are carrying yourself differently. Never wear a corset so tight that it restricts your breathing. A red face isn't sexy or healthy—nor is fainting. Wear it tight enough so you can feel it close to your skin but can still move around comfortably. A good test is to see whether you can pick something up from the floor while wearing it. You will notice that you move differently when you try this, as it will force you to bend your knees properly and keep your back straight. Have no doubt that you will draw more attention from the opposite sex—when you are ready for it (as you will be by the end of the program). You may discover a side to yourself you didn't know existed.

There are some fabulous Web sites that supply corsets and bustiers. You can find my favorite in the information section at the back of this book.

On the subject of underwear—please, please throw out your gray, baggy bras and panties. Nothing is more likely to maintain a negative self-image than bad underwear. If you would be embarrassed to be seen in public in them, don't wear them. Creating a feeling of sexiness by wearing beauti-ful underwear that fits you well will carry through to how you walk and stand—and you will find yourself smiling a lot more when you are in your sexy panties—I know I do.

## CARRY THAT LOAD

How often do you clear out your handbag? Or the bag you use for work, the rummage drawer in the kitchen, or the glove compartment of your car? Seriously—this is a real indicator of whether you are on top of things or they are on top of you. A friend had a handbag that was larger than the one I use for a weekend away: she was always running, always busy, forever stressed. I have known her since school, and knew that she had had a couple of rough times when she was growing up, and had turned into a typical overachiever. She only ever judged herself by her last piece of work or her children's ac-ademic results. Forever competing and vying for attention, it was as if she was afraid to stop because otherwise she would have to think about what she was doing. One day, when she was telling me just how miserable she was feeling about her weight, I noticed her huge handbag sitting beside her chair. I had never really realized it before, but she had taken to car-rying it everywhere with her, even when at home.

I took the bag, and weighed it. It weighed eight pounds—

the weight of four bags of sugar. It was only when she damaged her back picking up this load and she was laid up in bed that she finally took stock and looked at ways of reducing her load. She has since streamlined her handbag, her life—and her body. Clear out your bag every week—it takes a load off your mind as well as your shoulders.

## CONFIDENCE

All of the subjects in this chapter relate to confidence. Anything that will boost your confidence while you stay in control (so alcohol and drugs are out) is worth working on. Your confidence is the bedrock to creating and maintaining the changes that you want to make to your attitude, your body, yourself, and your weight.

Confidence will be yours when you are comfortable with your body—you already know that. Not when you reach a specific target, but when you start treating your body as if you like and value it—not as the enemy. Until then, and to help you get there faster, I have added suggestions into the third CD track to help you become more confident generally, and to disconnect the oversensitive connection between weight and confidence.

As you have worked your way through this book, listened to the CD, and completed the actions, you will have noticed your confidence increasing. *You will continue to become more confident in yourself, in your abilities, and in your feelings.* As your confidence grows, your focus on food will also change. *You will start to notice that you seem to have less time for snacks, you forget about eating by the clock, and you start to get fully engaged in whatever you are doing, to the complete exclusion of anything else.* Your attention now moves on to the world around you and the things that you can do to change your surroundings. This will have started with the small, practical measures of throwing away clothes that no longer fit you, and will have progressed to the more significant changes of letting go of thoughts and feelings that do not work for you anymore.

Your confidence is something to nurture and to care for. It is time now for you to be at the center of your universe, not your children, or your boss, or your partner—but you. You will notice that as a result of the changes that are happening— and will continue to strengthen over the next three weeks— you will feel much more assertive. And as you develop these skills and feelings you will notice when someone is trying to manipulate you. In the past you have grown used to being manipulated—by yourself—or more specifically, your negative self. This was the part of you who would persuade you to have that "extra cookie" or "just one more glass of wine." *This version of you is now a thing of the past, and you are left with skills that allow you to recognize immediately if someone else is trying to manipulate you emotionally.* This may be something of a revelation, and you might wonder why you did not notice this behavior from other people before. There are two reasons for this. One is that you were so involved with being manipulated by your negative self that you did not notice when someone else was doing it to you. The second reason is that when you take control of your body, your life, and your feelings about yourself, there will be other people around you who preferred you *as you were.* This is not because they are unpleasant people who want you to be miserable. These will be the people around you who care about you, and because of their own insecurities will want you back as you were *because that is who they felt comfortable with.* When you change and take control, you force other people around you to evaluate their own behavior.

Let me give you an example. I worked with a woman—let's call her Tara—who worked hard to lose weight but lacked the confidence and motivation to maintain the weight loss. She was a classic yo-yo dieter and would equate being slim with being happy. She had stories from her own life that, in her mind, proved this to be the case. She told me she only overate when she was unhappy. I pointed out the paradox in her statement. If she only overate when she was not happy, and she was only happy when she was slim—why did her weight yo-yo? Didn't that mean that at some point when she was slim, she would become unhappy and this is when she put the weight on? She recognized how odd this was, and when we worked this through, she recognized that there came a time during every slim phase when she started having massive arguments with her partner. He became very jealous, and if, say, she missed the bus home and was a few minutes late, he would accuse her of having an affair with someone at work whom she barely knew. He was unable to deal with her new, confident self, so he tried to change her back into the way she was before, when he knew how to deal with her.

Sometimes you have to recognize that it is other people's insecurities, not your own, that can become obstacles to real change. Once you recognize that it may not be *your* problem, or your fault that the arguments have started, then you can take a step back from them and allow yourself the space to change. If others can develop with you, then fine. If not, then you will find yourself changing more than your weight. You may realize that your relationship or your job have contributed to your weight gain. As a result of understanding yourself better you will also gain the confidence to make any other changes that need to happen in your life.

All changes have repercussions, and being confident will allow you to widen the scope of change in your life—and to take real control, once and for all.

## REAL TREATS

As you learn to take control of your feelings, and to respond to stress better, I believe that you deserve treats even more than before. It is very important that you decide what these treats are going to be, and create some new rituals to accommodate them.

I know that the idea of making an appointment with yourself may seem very artificial at first, but you will be surprised at how quickly you can get used to the idea. You schedule in visits to the dentist and doctors, don't you? So look on the *please yourself* time as maintenance. It will surprise you how quickly you start to look forward to this time. As for turning off your phone, you may be twitchy at first, but you will quickly get used to it. You are *not* on constant call unless this is a work requirement (and even in this situation it will not be *all* the time). Wean yourself away from responding to the phone without question, and never, ever answer your phone when you're eating. If one thing is guaranteed to create stress it is trying to have a conversation with someone while attempting to pay attention to your food. You are worth more than this. It is time for you to start respecting yourself in the way in which you would like other people to show respect to you.

The idea of treating yourself, and more significantly treat-

| Time Needed to Complete Action |  | 15 minutes |
| --- | --- | --- |

**ACTION**

Look at your diary and "book" an hour each week at the same time just for you.

Decide what you are going to do in that time.

Write it in there and make an appointment with yourself to *please yourself.*

If there are others in the house who claim your time, tell them that you are absolutely not to be disturbed. Even better, take yourself out of the house if you can.

*Turn off your phone.* Unless someone in the family or a close friend is seriously ill, there is no reason for your phone to be on constantly.

After three weeks of consistently keeping this appointment (and this is nonnegotiable), increase the time to two hours or two one-hour slots of *please yourself* time.

ing yourself *properly,* is an alien concept to most women—especially when they are feeling low or out of control. It is time for you to put yourself at the center of your world, where you belong. If the thought of doing this makes you nervous or stressed, then that is an indicator that you have not been looking after yourself properly for a long time. It can become a habit to put everyone else first, and the end result of this can be that you burn yourself out. The irony is that the people around you—those you *have* put first in your life—become so used to you doing everything for them that when you no longer can, because you have become so overwhelmed or ill, they don't know what to do to help you. They don't know how to do the things that you have done for them. Women will always be caregivers, and sometimes there is very little we can do to change this fact. However, when feeling insecure about ourselves we can sometimes confuse the attention given to us when we help others as love or affection—when in some instances we are actually being used by another person for their own benefit, and we choose not to notice it. You will have found suggestions in track two designed to put yourself in the center of your world and to let go of any guilt associated with taking care of yourself first. One of my favorite quotes from Shakespeare that I use in therapy with people who fall into this trap is *"Self-love is no vile a sin as self-neglect."* It is worth remembering.

Making space and time in your day to treat yourself sends out a message that you are important, and that you care about yourself. Why not start by organizing your beauty products? Throw away the ones that you have never used (and, be honest, never will use) and have cluttered up drawers and cupboards for ages (cosmetics do deteriorate) and put all the ones you will use in one place. Sort them into hair, body, and face products—then decide on a time and day when you are going to use them. I have my treat on Sunday night, as part of a bathing ritual. I feel all warm and pampered afterward, and there is nothing nicer than that groomed and indulged feeling. Believe me—you will get used to this and it will lift the way you feel.

Treats don't have to be expensive; it is about spending time and effort on yourself.

- Bathe away your stress.
- Give yourself a facial.
- Phone a friend.
- Listen to your favorite music.
- Read a book.
- Go for a long walk.

# FUTURE POSITIVE

YOU ARE COMING CLOSE TO THE END OF THE PROGRAM NOW, and this chapter contains the final hypnosis section—and it is one you will really enjoy. By listening to the third CD track when prompted, you will create and fix into your unconscious mind the future version of you that you can now imagine existing. Simply put, you are going to create your new self, as you will be when all the work you have done as part of this program is fully in place. This stage of the hypnotherapy will bring together everything you have learned or rejected on your way through the program. You will be in control now—making the decisions for yourself. You are now ready to make the changes happen—to make this new "self" the real, day-to-day living and breathing version of you.

How this will happen is interesting. I have already touched on how memories and future imaginings take place in the same part of the brain. In this section of the program we put this information to use by creating a future image of you that your unconscious mind will start to act on—as if it were already real. Your unconscious mind will not be able to distinguish whether the image is something that is still to happen, or has *already* happened. Therefore, when this future image is created, you will have something to look *forward* to and to *reflect* upon. This means that you can start afresh with the new version of you—adding characteristics and traits that you have never had before. You will be the person you have always wanted to be, but never *really* believed you could become.

*This new version of you will be self-confident and attractive, assertive and positive.* The *new* self that you are about to become will be able to get excited about life and future possibilities, instead of constantly looking back into the past. Most important of all, the version of you that you are about to create will no longer be obsessed with weight. When the obsession is gone, then all the stress associated with it will leave as well. The weight will naturally leave with it, and your new self will move into successful patterns of behavior that will not only get you where you want to be with your life but also help you to remain at a weight that feels natural and healthy *for you.*

In the last hypnosis track at the end of this chapter, you will be prompted to visualize your future self. When this happens, it doesn't matter if you cannot consciously access an image.

Your unconscious mind begins to motivate you to stay on track. Your future self will say, "No, don't eat that doughnut. You have that dress to fit into." "Think about what people will say when you walk through that door looking fabulous."

The process of creating your future, positive self will happen *unconsciously*—without you being aware that it is happening. When you allow your unconscious mind to do this, it works much better than thinking about how you want to be. This is because people are very good at talking themselves out of change—but when this process is unconscious, *all you notice is that you are changing and improving each day*—not *how* it happens.

Sometimes our unconscious mind will protect us from information that it feels we cannot, at this moment, accept. This is for our own good. Recognize that this is a natural process that has happened before, and will happen again. You will, however, start to meet your new self in your dreams. *Listen to this final track*—Future—*for the next twenty-one nights.*

*During this time you will be familiarizing yourself with the person you are about to reveal to the world. You will make the image of your future self strong enough to start driving your new, positive behaviors.*

You will soon start to trust your unconscious mind fully when you notice the new thoughts, feelings, and behaviors that filter through to your day-to-day awareness as a result.

## LIVING IN THE PRESENT

Our brain has a phenomenal capacity to allow our mental landscape to move through time. With this ability, we can remember what we were doing on our twenty-first birthday and how we felt, and we can imagine how we are going to experience a holiday we have not yet had. This ability to predict the future is primarily connected with our facility for remembering past events. The same areas of the brain are involved in remembering (past) and imagining (future). The implications of this are phenomenal in terms of making long-term changes to any aspect of your life. In relation to changing how you feel about your body and your relationship with food, making the appropriate connections between your memory and your imagination will completely alter your future relationship with your body. Most important, it will allow for variations. This means that if, in the future, your body changes—whether it is through pregnancy or life change—you will accommodate this change and it will not have a negative impact on how you view yourself. You will not constantly refer to a past "fixed" image of yourself as an ideal, or strive for something that is not going to be possible to change.

The program in this book, particularly the CD component, works by activating useful and positive associations that then form the basis of new neurological connections. These connections are reinforced by reading this book, and carrying out the activities in each chapter. This will create a strong, confident image to build upon. You do not need to do or think anything more, but you will start to notice the changes as they happen to you.

How you responded to the suggestions in the earlier hypnosis tracks depended initially on how you related to your history. There are two ways that this can affect our relationship with our bodies. There are those individuals who have had the balance right at some time in their life—and there are those who have never (or at least feel that they have never) been comfortable with their bodies or in their relationship with food.

The former group will have found this program easier, as it contained a sequence of suggestions that they could disregard. If you are in the second group, and feel that you cannot

## CASE | STUDIES

### HOW YOUR PAST AFFECTS HOW YOU
### RESPOND TO THE PROGRAM

Christine had never felt good about herself or her weight. She needed to develop confidence and self-esteem before she was going to be able to make the changes necessary to take control of her weight. As she worked her way through the program, she noticed that she started to feel better about herself and generally more in control even though she hadn't yet lost any weight. However, once she recognized that she had more control over the things that used to stress her, she then felt strong enough to make the changes needed to lose weight.

Anita, on the other hand, had only put weight on when pregnant with her first child, and she hadn't lost it by the time she had her second. She was feeling fat and frumpy, but unlike Christine she could remember a time when she had felt good about her weight. She responded to the suggestions for change almost immediately, and the image of herself as she had been before the pregnancies motivated her to stick to the program.

For Christine, she had to create a confident self—Anita just needed to reconnect with it. This is why for some of us the process takes longer to start than others.

remember a time when you were happy with yourself or your weight, then there was a whole set of suggestions that were the key to long-term change for you. One of the most wonderful things, I feel, about allowing your unconscious mind to do the work for you is that you do not need to think too hard about the process; just allow it to work *with* you.

## TAKING CONTROL OF YOUR ATTITUDES TOWARD FOOD AND YOUR CURRENT SELF

Ever since you listened to the first CD track, unconscious changes have been taking place. You probably won't have noticed yet, but by the time you have finished this book you will recognize that you have a different attitude toward yourself and the world around you. *You will feel better, more optimistic, and more relaxed—above all, you will be ready to get on with doing all the things you already know will work for you so you can lose weight forever.*

Along the way you will have noticed that some of the sections have made complete sense to you, as if you always knew these things (even if you couldn't always put them into practice). You may have found yourself skimming through these sections. And there may have been others that were all new to you, with concepts that took a little time to absorb—not just because they were new, but also because they were about your feelings and how you relate to yourself as an individual. You will have noticed that with some of the suggestions, whether in the book or on the CD, you did not feel the desire to spend too much time absorbing this information, and there may have been some that you positively rejected. If this is the case, fine. Remember the 80/20 rule I talked about earlier. You only need to take on board one suggestion in five for the process to work effectively for you.

## SCARE YOURSELF—THROW OFF YOUR FEAR OF CHANGE

Changing can be scary; many of us cling to the old and familiar rather than face the scary feelings that can accompany change. This program will help you to embrace that fear and welcome change.

The way to do this is to get your adrenaline going. It is time to get excited at the real possibilities of how your life is going to change when you have control over your weight. If the thought of doing something scares you, then your heart rate rises, increasing your metabolism and pushing up your blood sugar level—giving you a rush. If you are bored with your life and the world around you, you will get your sugar rush from a tin—the cookie tin. There is no excuse for doing this from now on, because the hypnotherapy suggestions you have already listened to will be taking effect. Any sensations that you used to associate with fear (shortness of breath, sweaty palms, butterflies in your stomach) you can now start to associate with excitement. Fear and excitement are the same on a physical level, and the hypnosis suggestions that excite you will allow you to experience these sensations and interpret them in a new way—as something to welcome.

Excite yourself by embracing the fear of change by doing something differently. Research has shown that if you do one thing a day that increases your adrenaline (in other words something that scares you), you will lose weight without making any other changes.

You should now be getting enthusiastic about the possibility of a real change in your life, one that will give you back the control and the confidence you need to change your weight and your life forever.

## WHEN I LOSE WEIGHT I WILL . . .

In your quest to free yourself from your body obsession and the damaging effects of yo-yo dieting, you will probably have experienced times when you daydreamed of how your life was going to be when you had lost the weight and gained control over your eating habits. For instance, when I lose weight I will:

- have a good relationship
- be happy
- get the job I want
- leave my partner
- write a book
- move

You can add just about any goal you want here. Postponing success can be a major reason for getting stuck in the status quo of our relationship with our bodies—which means staying unhappy. This is all about making choices. If you have ever found yourself thinking about how different your life could be when you lost weight, I want you to remember that the ability to make those changes is not directly connected to your weight. If they were, nobody who identified themselves as having a weight problem would ever have achieved anything in their lives. When we postpone our future it is because we do not have the confidence to change. For some of us, this is because body confidence and the confidence to do other things in our lives *have* become inextricably linked. Some of the suggestions in the final hypnosis track will break down this unnatural connection, so that your confidence to do other things in your life will grow as the link between your body image and your confidence diminishes. There are other suggestions on the track designed to replace these unwanted connections by building confidence and developing feelings of self-esteem.

As a result of the hypnosis you will set and achieve a series of small, realistic goals. A habit of success will develop in you so that changing and developing will become habitual and will grow to feel completely natural. Being at ease with yourself should not have to be a conscious effort. The hypnosis will help move the changes into your unconscious processes as quickly and easily as possible—and as your confidence grows, so will the size of your goals that you will unconsciously set as you continue with the CD after you've finished this book. Change will become a comfortable habit.

## BROADEN YOUR EMOTIONAL HORIZONS

It can be so much easier to feel sorry for ourselves when we are feeling overweight than to get out there and interact with other people. As we become more self-absorbed and miserable, it is too easy to forget that there are so many people who do not have a fraction of what we have. When we feel unhappy about our weight we become self-obsessed and closed off. When I work one-to-one with individuals, I encourage them as part of the process of change to sponsor a child through Plan International, or a woman through Women for Women (a charity that sponsors women who have been victims of war). By direct sponsorship of another individual, your focus of attention moves away from yourself, and you can start to redirect those feelings into something more positive.

This may seem harsh, but moving your focus away from yourself will give you a completely different perspective on your problems. You will soon gain a different sense of balance. I started doing this for myself and I soon discovered that it is almost impossible to feel sorry for myself. No matter what happens, I am still better off than most of the population of this planet. We have choices. Part of this program is about exercising those choices to give ourselves the life we want—and if someone you have never met benefits through your process of change, it is all for the best.

So go and volunteer. Help repair stone walls in Yorkshire, clear canal banks in London, or whatever interests you. Go on a volunteering holiday. You will find the details in the useful contacts at the end of this book. When you volunteer you remove yourself from your usual routine, making a real difference not only to your body but also to your environment.

## SLOW DOWN

Eat more slowly. We all know we should, but I wonder if you are aware of how many fast-food outlets design their furniture, music, and lighting to unconsciously influence you to eat more quickly. Eating fast becomes a habit, almost a badge of honor for some people, as if it is some indicator of how efficient they are. The fact is, when we eat more slowly we digest more efficiently, feel full sooner, and therefore eat less. It is not only the fast-food outlets that are aware of this. Many ready-made foods are packaged in "bite-size" chunks, so they can be eaten quickly. The texture of most of these foods is also such that you don't have to chew too hard or too much. Baby food, in other words—sweet and soft and weirdly satisfying. It appeals to the helpless child within us. As you take control of yourself and your feelings about your body, your tastes will mature, and you will want something with a bit more "bite," more variety and texture, more flavor. This will be true not only for your food but will extend into your other tastes as well.

Life is about pleasure—or so it should be. If you have ever experienced severe illness, or lost someone close to you, you know how it changes the way you respond to the world around you. A couple of years ago I found that I was unable to look after myself after a back injury. I could read, but not for long. I could write, but quickly lost concentration. I was bedridden and very quickly became incredibly bored. After a week or so, I started to notice different things. The scent of the pineapple in the fruit basket that a friend had sent to me seemed to fill the room, and I, who never ate fruit before, could smell the scents of the different fruits in turn. My whole mouth turned to liquid, and all I wanted to do was eat that fruit. I couldn't reach it, though, and by the time someone came to help me, I fell on that fruit as if it was the only thing in the world I had ever wanted.

When you are ill, your world becomes narrow and you begin to notice things that other people do not even register. What I am attempting to get across here is that it is the small things in life that are important, things that we often overlook in our self-obsessed race to wherever we are going.

Being thin does not *make* you happy, nor does being rich— *you make you happy,* and you do this by appreciating the simple things. Time on the phone with someone you care about, a walk in the countryside—simple pure pleasures—not money and a stick-thin, unhealthy body.

## A RITUAL TO SAY GOOD-BYE

The next step in this process is to make space for a new and confident look for the new you.

It is time now to make the commitment to moving on. You will have to make an appointment in your diary to say good-bye to those comfortable disguises that no longer have a place in your life. You will need a whole day to do this. Book it now. I know this sounds odd—and a little dramatic, perhaps, but physically clearing out the wardrobe is more than a spring cleaning.

This process of clearing out can be emotional. If you have a good friend you can call on to help, that's even better. You will be amazed at the conversations this will prompt if you do—especially when your friend starts to tell you what they thought about the person you were when you were wearing those clothes. You will realize how different you were when you wore them, and how people responded to you as a different person. In terms of how people relate to you, you are what you wear.

Do not continue with the program until you have made this commitment with yourself. Only then can you continue with this book. On the morning of the day that you have allocated to do this task, read on.

When you have done this, I want you to take a moment and remember why you did it. Whether the clothes were cheap or expensive, whether you bought them or were given them as gifts, it doesn't matter now. The only thing that matters is that you are clearing the way for your new, confident self—and there will be no going back, only forward.

Now it is time for you to listen to the third and final track on the CD. Creating a template of how you will *feel* when you have finished the program is just as important as creating an

| Time Needed to Complete Action |  | 4 to 6 hours |
| --- | --- | --- |

**ACTION**

Go to your wardrobe and empty it completely. I mean everything—just as if you were moving.

Put the clothes into piles by type: shoes together, pants together, skirts together, handbags all together. Use different rooms of the house if you need to until you have everything sorted.

Make two piles:

- Charity shop
- Keep

You will need to repeat this action with the clothes in your drawers, chests, under the bed, and anywhere else you have been storing clothes.

*Remember*—your underwear counts as clothing too!

Take the bags to the charity shop straightaway if you can. If not, put them by the door ready to go.

Everything that is staying, you can now return to the wardrobe, drawers, and cupboards. You will have plenty of room to organize it logically so you can see where everything is.

## HYPNOSIS | SESSION 3

**THE FUTURE**

| Time Needed to Complete Action | ⏱ | 30 minutes |
|---|---|---|

**ACTION**

Track three: *Future*

Go to the toilet if you need to.

Turn off your phone and minimize any possible distractions.

Choose a time and find a place where you can be undisturbed. You can sit down or lie down, as long as you are comfortable. Do not cross your arms or legs; allow them to relax.

If you wear glasses, take them off.

Close your eyes.

Now listen to the third track on the CD, called *Future*.

When the track is over, sit or lie still for a few moments to make sure you are fully reoriented.

*Remember:* if anything happens that requires your attention while you are listening to the CD, you will become fully alert and able to respond.

image of how you will look. The feelings that you are about to generate in the third and final hypnosis track will be ones that will keep you from slipping back into old patterns of behavior. You will learn to trust these feelings, too, and understand that even if you feel slightly uncomfortable the first time you exercise them (for example, the first time you are assertive and say no to a situation that in the past you automatically said yes to), you will very quickly notice the benefits of this new behavior, and it will become more comfortable and safe for you in future.

# WELCOMING THE NEW YOU

YOU HAVE NOW LISTENED TO ALL THREE TRACKS ONCE AND that completes the first stage of the hypnotherapy. The second and final stage ends when you have listened to track three for twenty-one days in total.

If, at any point from then on, you feel you need a boost, you can listen to track three again. Forget about tracks one and two; you have now finished with them. This final chapter pulls together all the themes in the program. Your past, present, and future are now where they should be. Your unconscious mind has been given all the information it needs.

You will start feeling much more motivated and positive, and you will look forward to the changes as they happen.

## MORE THAN CLOTHES . . . YOUR NEW PERSONALITY

Throughout this program you may have recognized that the suggestions that I have made were all designed so that you could follow them with small, manageable steps. We started by changing the quick and simple things, and by doing the easiest first, you have built up your stamina for change and created a habit of change that will spread into other areas of your life. Now that you are close to the end of this book I want to tell you something that you were not ready to hear before. *You are a remarkable and unique individual.* Everything you have known and experienced makes you who you are today—a very special person. You have used this program to create a fresh, new you, and you built it up from within yourself. Long-term change comes about when you accept that you are responsible for the person you have become, and then can set about changing who you are, and how you are seen by other people.

You are now ready to meet a slimmed-down version of yourself. A new, strong, definite version of you is here, and you can now take the final action, which will send you on your way to becoming the person you have always wanted to be.

After listening to the final hypnosis track, your unconscious is now ready to make the slimmed-down version of you a reality. I want you to take a moment to rest before you do anything else.

You may now find that you have hardly any clothes left, so it is time to go shopping. Go and shop for the new you. You know what will look good on you—now that you have one, confident self, you can start to listen to your own inner, encouraging voice. If you would like a little help then, treat yourself to a personal shopper. Most department stores have them and, contrary to popular belief, you do not *have* to buy. You will find that the act of spending time with someone else who is interested in you looking good will be great for your confidence anyway, and you will come away with information on shapes and styles that are right for you.

Or perhaps you have already read enough magazines, looked at enough catalogs, and seen enough programs telling you how to dress to impress, which makes you quite an expert when you think about it. It's time to get out there and dress your new character. When you see her in the changing room mirror smiling back at you, you will know that you are a different person. Even if you do not buy the clothes there and then—even if you are only taking her out for a test run—she is starting to emerge from the cocoon of those old selves. Never again keep something "for best." Today is the day to wear those clothes. Today is going to be the best day for you,

because you are now able to step into the shoes (and the clothes) of your new self.

## The Reveal

Do you remember playing dress-up as a kid? Now is the time to dress up as your new self.

## PREPARE FOR WHO YOU ARE GOING TO BE TOMORROW

There are still a few loose ends to tie up so that you maintain the progress you have made as part of the program. The

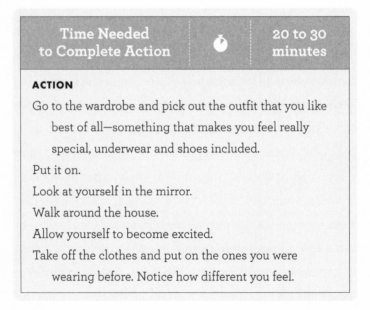

| Time Needed to Complete Action | ⏱ | 20 to 30 minutes |
| --- | --- | --- |

**ACTION**

Go to the wardrobe and pick out the outfit that you like best of all—something that makes you feel really special, underwear and shoes included.

Put it on.

Look at yourself in the mirror.

Walk around the house.

Allow yourself to become excited.

Take off the clothes and put on the ones you were wearing before. Notice how different you feel.

biggest one of these involves your changing some of your habits. You have worked on the way you think, feel, and behave—but habits are different and need to be dealt with separately. To further clarify the difference: habits are what we do automatically without thought; behaviors are the actions we take.

If your habit is to get up in the morning and root through the wardrobe to see what is clean/handy/comfortable without putting much thought into it, you will be unconsciously re-acting to "first morning thoughts." Already you have started to change those thoughts, but even if you have changed those "It's going to be a rotten day today" or "Nothing special is going on today" thoughts, you are still in the habit of dressing accordingly. There is a way in which you can get around this until you develop the new habit of giving yourself positive suggestions for the day. There is a simple, practical strategy that involves deciding who you are going to be tomorrow *the night before.*

Before you get into bed, lay out the clothes you are going to wear tomorrow, including underwear and shoes. This is a good habit to get into even when you have got your daily mind-set sorted out. It reduces the stress of finding clothes when you are tired, and it also means that by handling the clothes in which you are expecting to have a good day, you are creat-ing positive tactile associations with those clothes. You will start to associate having a good time with the feel of those clothes as well as their look. I have a bright orange velvet scarf at home—and whenever I stroke it, it makes me smile. I remember having some wonderful, happy experiences when I was wearing it. The clothes belonging to the new, positive self will have these associations, because you will create them—just as you created negative associations with some of the clothes you used to wear.

By laying out your clothes the night before you are allowing your unconscious mind to prepare mentally for the day ahead. I can give you a lovely example. I got married recently—and on the eve of my wedding, my beautiful dress was hanging in the bedroom with me. I found myself looking at it, imagining how I was going to feel wearing it. Now the dress has been made into a textile sculpture that hangs on my wall, and every time I see it I remember the wonderful feelings I experienced on that day.

Obviously, that was a very special day for me, but you can make any day as special as possible. When you know what you are going to wear the next day, your dreams start to include *how you are going to feel in those clothes*—and how other people are going to react to you when you are wearing them. The clothes you plan to wear are all part of planning the type of day you are going to have. As you start doing this, you begin to recognize that every day can be special—because you make it that way.

It is wonderful when other people start to notice the changes in you, and you will be amazed how many people think that you have lost weight already because they can see more of your shape—or think that you have a new lover.

## TURN OFF THE TELEVISION

When I was a kid, there was a program on TV in which the theme tune included the words, "Why don't you turn off your TV set and do something less boring instead?" Even as a child I was aware of the irony of a television program that encouraged us not to watch TV. It seems that many of us who grew up with this are quite content to live our lives vicariously through reality TV. Thinking of moving? Watch a program about it. Living abroad? We have the show for you. Want to feel that you have friends? Watch Big Brother. John Lennon said, "Life is what happens while you're busy making other plans." Postponing the start of your life until something magical happens does not work—you will just get older, more fixed in your thinking, and less likely to do something about it.

What I am trying to get across to you is that the only time

to make those changes to your life is now. The best time to take control is now—not next week or next month—now. This is where the mental tricks that you have played on yourself up until this point end. Forget about TV programs that tell you how to live your life. It is time to move from remote control to real control—control of your life. The program that you have now experienced through reading, completing the actions, and listening to the CD will give you that control, allowing you to *live your life free from the guilt and confusion of your history.*

You will live more easily in the present, looking forward to your future while being conscious of your habits and being able to embrace change.

## FUTURE POSSIBILITIES

As we near the end of the program, I would like to remind you of something you have probably done before, and reassure you that this time—probably for the first time—you are *not* going to fall into the old trap. In the past you have probably read books, listened to CDs, and watched DVDs about fitness and health. In some instances, you may even have tried to copy what you have seen or heard. Then, after a couple of weeks you noticed that you kept finding other things to do instead of incorporating your newly discovered knowledge into your life. For example, a year ago, I decided to clear out some books, videos, and other odds and ends to take to the charity shop. What I discovered was a veritable historical record of obsession with the shape of my body. Fitness balls and bands, books on calisthenics (does anyone remember that?), videos with Jane Fonda, and there was *lots* of stuff that I could not remember buying, using, or—more important—benefiting from. I got rid of the lot. All of that equipment and information just served to remind me of one thing—until I worked on my mind I had failed my body.

This program has worked for me, and for many clients who came to me with a body issue. It is a simple equation—get your head straight using hypnotherapy, and your attitude toward your body and your self will straighten out *automatically*. Diet and exercise are not the key. Getting a mind-set that will let you take care of your body properly, and doing the things that you already know you ought to be doing—that is the key to long-term physical and emotional health.

This time you have no more excuses. I have taken you through all the reasons *why* you have had problems before, and by using the hypnosis have given you suggestions that you can now take on board unconsciously. Most important of all, I have helped you work on and develop the confidence and self-belief that you will now use to motivate yourself. As I said at the start of the book, no one can make you do anything you don't want to do. From this point in time that includes you. You will no longer be able to trick or fool yourself again when it comes to food, exercise, and attitude. The hypnotherapy that you have experienced stops this mind game from happening. The only suggestions you will listen to, from yourself, are those that will move you closer to your goals. You may even find it annoying at times, but that's just tough. This is your unconscious mind speaking, so listen up. No more opportunity to postpone success—you simply have to get on with it, right now.

What will be interesting, and you will notice if it happens, is when other people try to pull you back into your old way of thinking and doing things. This is simply because they are stuck in the rut you used to be in. These are the women who go to the gym but persuade you to go in the Jacuzzi instead of having a swim. These are the friends who say they will come for a walk with you tomorrow and then find an excuse when you call for them. You will notice it, and it will make you smile—especially when they see how you have changed (for the better), and they ask you what your secret is. You will deal with these situations by being even more motivated and confident. You are in control now and you will really notice how much better it feels.

## FUTURE RECALL

The preparation for change is almost complete, and you are almost ready to set out on your journey of change. Before going anywhere, however, it is important to know where you are going, and this is a fundamental aspect to obtaining and maintaining positive feelings about yourself and your body. Seeing yourself in the outfit is a start. Feeling those clothes on your skin and allowing yourself to get excited is the next step. Remember, if you do not decide *how* you want to be when you have changed, then how are you going to know when you have succeeded? Playing dress-up is the beginning.

Accept that before any external change can be made, and the neurological connections stimulated sufficiently to build new and effective habits for your future, you will need to recognize the internal image of yourself, *as you will be when the change has occurred*. In other words, you will have a new template of yourself. This has been created in the hypnosis based on what you want from your future, not borrowed from your past. It takes around three weeks for you to really get to grips with this new self, and until then you will feel as if you are acting, and that the new version of you is not quite real. It isn't—yet. Only when the three weeks is over—and you have had twenty-one nights of sleep—only then will the new image be strong enough to allow you to forget about it, consciously. It will become an unconscious self that is strong and able to deal with anything, anybody, and any situation. This emotionally healthy and stable version of you is flexible and has stamina—and is here to stay no matter what.

## TREAT YOURSELF BETTER

There will always be times for celebrations and treats—birthdays, weddings, holidays. Enjoy these times and cut yourself some slack. It is perfectly okay to put on a little weight when you are on holiday—and to lose it gradually when you come home. It is fine to have that piece of cake on your birthday, or even have a blowout and drink much more than you would normally imbibe. This program is not about restriction—it is about recognizing that life is all about variety. Without the celebrations there would be very little joy in life.

I made suggestions in the second hypnosis track designed to help you let go of the guilt that you have in the past associated with having a good time and letting your hair down, and suggestions in the third track for being flexible about life in general and food in particular. When you enjoy life to the fullest, your unconscious can begin to learn that variety is good. It is not healthy to always restrict yourself—you put your body into starvation mode and it holds on to every bit of fat that comes its way. When you allow yourself to enjoy life, your unconscious can learn that there will always be food available for you and will send out hunger signals that you can recognize and will respond to appropriately. You will eat in response to true hunger—and enjoy it.

A very different set of mental connections has happened now that the effects of the program are kicking in. Your unconscious mind starts to learn that you can enjoy yourself, and will accommodate your behavior after this point so that you can cut back on your intake as a way of balancing out the indulgence. The difference takes effect when the guilt of pleasure is removed. All the work you have done on your past self and on your present now takes effect in helping you to recognize on both a conscious and an unconscious level that you are allowed to have fun. You are in control, and the balance that you have been working toward is now taking hold.

You will start to notice as the days and the weeks and the months go by that you have stopped worrying about the celebration times, and you have instead started to look forward to them. Your body now prepares to metabolize the food you are about to eat at the party in a completely different way. As you now allow yourself to get excited about the idea of a celebration (rather than dreading it as you used to), you are producing adrenaline, and the speed of your metabolism is increasing. Increased anticipation—increased excitement—increased rate of digestion for the food you are about to eat. Simple. Look forward to your celebrations and you create a system ready to process that food more rapidly. Instead of dread feel anticipation. Instead of guilt, feel pleasure. You are changing more than your attitude toward your body—*you are now truly changing your mind.*

## SADNESS—DISTRACTION

Just as there are times to have fun and to celebrate life, there are times when we get sad. If for you sadness and eating have been connected, you will now recognize how dangerous this can be, as the sadness trigger can spiral into a binge that then brings on guilt, disgust, and more sadness at your apparent inability to control yourself.

It is an unalterable fact—sad things occur in life. We feel that sadness, and that is appropriate. It is healthy to allow yourself to feel and to express sadness. What is *not* appropriate for someone who has comfort eaten in the past is to be *unthinking* at the time of sadness, because this can allow the habits of comfort eating to move into action. To help prevent this, I have embedded something called an "anchor" as part of the second hypnosis track, and it is designed to be used when something makes you feel sad. In fact, the anchor can be used when any emotion occurs that used to trigger your negative behaviors. The really nice thing about using anchors to help you break negative patterns is that once they are in place they will happen automatically—without your even being aware that something has triggered them. An anchor is a physical movement (in this instance, gently squeezing the left-hand edge of the wrist on your right hand with the thumb and first finger of your left hand). It will help. I chose this particular movement as an anchor because as well as helping you to find and lock in positive feelings it is also an acupressure point called *Shen-man,* meaning "divine gate." In acupressure, putting gentle pressure on this point calms the mind when it is overactive and you're thinking too much, relieves anxiety and sleeplessness, and creates a feeling of peace. By learning this anchor while you are in hypnosis and feeling relaxed, you will be able to bring this feeling to yourself whenever you need it. Remember, the pressure is a gentle one.

## THREE WEEKS ON—ONE WEEK OFF

Whenever you are trying to create a new habit or pattern for yourself, it is important to understand the two main components that influence long-term change. First, it takes three weeks to build a habit—twenty-one nights of sleep during which time your REM sleep turns the changes from conscious acts into unconscious processes. Second, a period of rest needs to be built into the pattern for it to become long-lasting. This rest period is *essential*. It gives you time to allow the new habits to settle in before you take on any more changes, while at the same time allowing you to refine the changes—to make them your own. If you try to make long-term changes to your behaviors without the rest period you may quickly find that stress occurs and you will "fall off the wagon" somehow. You will overeat or find an excuse not to exercise—then you find that you are talking yourself into seeing this as a failure. Most people who have tried to take control of their weight at some point in their lives recognize this danger sign. It is as if a negative version of yourself takes over and reminds you that *"this is what always happens"* or *"it's not fair, I have been good all week."* Recognize it? This is the part of you that knows that you need time off from any change plan. But it does not have the capacity to switch the good habit back on. You can forget about this; I made suggestions on the CD that will help you do two things in relation to this. First, they will help you to switch on the rest time and then switch back on the program at the end of that rest. Second, the suggestions will help you to recognize the negative version of yourself that reared up in the past—and turn it off immediately.

By following this "three weeks on, one week off" framework you will work with your body, not against it. If you are

WELCOMING THE NEW YOU

a woman of childbearing age, use your period as the time for rest. The rest of you can choose when you want your rest time to occur. The key to this is that it has to be regular and consistent. There is no point saying to yourself, "The program is so easy that I won't need the rest period—I can just continue with what I am doing." You can't—so don't try. You will find that you settle very quickly into this new pattern of "three weeks on, one week off." This will happen because it feels natural—and it is. Nature works on these cycles, so whether you are an athlete training for a race or a crop farmer working your fields, there is a natural requirement to make time for rest. The mental work necessary to turn this program into new habits for life still continues even though you are physically doing nothing. Enjoy it—it is a necessary part of the cycle.

The work has now been done. All that remains is for you to allow the changes to become habits. During the next three weeks, all I want you to do is *notice* what you are doing differently. It may feel like a lot or a little, but the most important thing for you to know is that during the next three weeks your unconscious mind is processing everything you have read and listened to. This will happen at night, when you sleep and when you dream. As the days go by, you will notice that things that you are doing differently that at first seemed like an effort will no longer be apparent to you as you start to do them habitually. The program was designed to replicate natural patterns of learning and development, and as such it should at no point feel as if you have dramatically changed. Look back on yourself three months from the end of this book, however, and you will see a new person looking back at you, a person who is confident, happy, and well on track for an exciting future.

I hope that you have enjoyed this process of finding the real, in-control you, and now appreciate what you've found in yourself. The process you started by doing this program doesn't end here or in three weeks or three months. Your change and development is now an ongoing event—a program in itself. By working on yourself you have now created a habit that actually has very little to do with your weight, but one that will allow you to weigh your choices differently and find a balance in life that will work better for you. Your new habit is one of feeling good about yourself. As you present yourself differently, people will react differently to you. Here's to being a whole new person. Congratulations. It's time to get hold of life with both hands and be the person that wonderful things happen to. After all the work that you have done, you will look for happiness, find it—and deserve it.

Love life.

Best wishes, Ursula James

# USEFUL WEB ADDRESSES

### HYPNOTHERAPY SESSIONS, CDS, BOOKS, AND COURSES

www.ursulajames.com

### VOLUNTEERING HOLIDAYS

www.ethicalvolunteering.org

www.goabroad.com

www.responsibletravel.com

### CORSETS AND BUSTIERS

www.victoriassecret.com

### COUNSELING AND PSYCHOTHERAPY

American Association for Marriage and Family Therapy

www.aamft.com

American Psychological Association

www.apa.org

## ORGANIC FRUIT AND VEGETABLES

www.wholefoodsmarket.com

## WORKSHOPS AND COURSES

Ursula runs one-day "You can think yourself thin" workshops throughout the year. You can find details at www.ursula james.com and follow the link for training.

You can also contact the author at books@ursulajames.com.